PALEO DIET FOR ATHLETES AND SPORTSMEN

COMPLETE GUIDE AND COOKBOOK FOR ATHLETES AND SPORTSMEN WHO WANT TO FOLLOW THE PALEO DIET TO GET FIT AND REGULATE THEIR WEIGHT

(200 RECIPES)

By

Jack HARRIS

TABLE OF CONTENS

INTRODUCTION TO PALEO DIET FOR ATHLETES AND SPORTSMEN

This book contains a specific guide and cookbook for athletes and sportsmen and women who want to follow the Paleo Diet, maintain a healthy diet and regulate their weight. There are 200 easy-to-make, original, delicious and appetising recipes that will help you follow the diet plan.

BENEFITS OF PALEO DIET

The paleo diet plan is a diet program that mimics how pre-historic people could have eaten. It entails consuming whole food items that people could search for or collect. Promoters from the paleo diet plan decline new diet programs that are usually filled with processed food items. They think that time for how hunter- gatherers consumed could cause fewer health issues. The paleo diet plan isn't safe for everybody. Physicians have no idea of its results on kids, women that are pregnant, or old grownups. Individuals with persistent problems, such as inflammatory intestinal illness, should talk to a physician before trying a paleo diet plan. This manual explores paleo principles, and a 7-day paleo diet meal intends to follow. Please continue reading to understand how to consume like our forefathers. The paleo diet plan's focus is on eating foodstuffs that might have already been obtainable in the Paleolithic era. Furthermore, the paleo diet plan will be referred to as the rock age group diet plan, hunter-gatherer diet plan, or caveman diet plan. Before contemporary agriculture developed around 10,000 years back, people usually ate foods they could hunt or gather, such as fish, liver organs, fruits, vegetables, peanuts, and seeds. The introduction of modern farming changed how people ate. Milk products, dried beans, and grains grew to become a section of people's diet plans. Advocates from the paleo diet plan believe that the body hasn't evolved to procedure dairy products, dried beans, and grains that feed on these food types could raise the threat of specific health issues, such as cardiovascular disease, being overweight, and diabetes.

HEALTH ADVANTAGES OF PALEO

Individuals declare that the paleo diet plan gives numerous health advantages, such as promoting weight reduction, reducing the chance of diabetes, and ecreasing blood pressure. In this area, we go through the scientific evidence to find out what the study facilitates these claims:

EXCESS WEIGHT LOSS

A mature 2008 research discovered that 14 healthy volunteers achieved the average weight reduction of 2.3 kilos by following a paleo diet plan for three weeks. In 2009, researchers compared the paleo diet plan's consequences with the diet plan for diabetes on 13 people with type 2 diabetes. Little research discovered that consuming the paleo method decreased individuals' body weight and waistline area. The 2014 research of 70 post-menopausal ladies with weight problems discovered that carrying out a paleo diet plan helped individuals shed weight after six months. Nevertheless, right after 24 months, there has been simply no difference in weight reduction among individuals following a paleo diet and the ones sticking with regular Nordic nutritional suggestions. These outcomes claim that some other healthy diet programs could be as effective at advertising weight reduction.

The authors of the 2017 review noted that this paleo diet plan helped reduce weight for a while but figured this result is because of caloric restriction or consuming fewer calories. Generally, the study shows that the paleo diet plan can help people shed weight initially, but that additional diet plans that reduce calorie consumption might be effective. Even more, the study is essential before physicians recommend the paleo diet plan for weight reduction. Presently, physicians recommend visitors to follow a calorie- controlled exercise and diet even more to lose excess weight

REDUCING THE RISK OF DIABETES

Does following a Paleo diet program reduce the risk of diabetes? The results of some preliminary research are usually encouraging. Insulin resistance is a dangerous element in the development of diabetes. Improving a person's sensitivity to insulin levels reduces the likelihood that it can lead to diabetes and helps those who have diabetes to reduce their symptoms. A 2015 study compared the consequences of a Paleo diet plan to the consequences of a diet plan predicted by the recommendations of your American Diabetes Association on people who have type 2 diabetes. While both diet programs improved the metabolic health of individuals, the paleo diet plan improved insulin resistance and blood sugar control. A 2009 study of nine sedentary volunteers without obesity found that the Paleo diet plan improved insulin awareness. There is a requirement for a more recent study for the paleo diet plan and diabetes. However, the evidence to date suggests that a hunter-gatherer-like diet may improve insulin sensitivity.

REDUCING BLOOD PRESSURE

Elevated blood pressure is a prospective factor in cardiovascular disease. Many people believe that a paleo diet plan can help keep blood pressure in balance and promote coronary heart health. Research conducted in 2008 on 14 healthy volunteers found that following a paleo diet plan for 3 weeks improved systolic blood pressure. In addition, overweight and whole-body body mass index (BMI) decreased. The analysis does not add handle to the team, and yet, the results are usually not conclusive. Research from 2014 supported these early results. Experts compared the consequences of a Paleo diet plan with the consequences of a diet plan recommended by Dutch wellness authorities on 34 individuals with traits of metabolic symptoms, a disorder that increases the danger of cardiovascular disease. The outcomes showed how the Paleo diet plan lowered the users' blood pressure and bloodstream lipid profile, which may improve wellness centers. Although preliminary studies claim that the Paleo diet can lower blood pressure and promote heart health, newer and larger studies are needed to draw conclusions.

HOW TO START A DIET

The Paleo diet will supposedly rid you of migraines, eliminate bloating, eliminate seasonal allergies, clear up acne, and shed a few pounds. While none of this is guaranteed, cleaning up your diet and focusing on fresh, wholesome foods is a good idea. Natural foods in reasonable portions will help you feel reasonably satisfied because they help maintain your blood sugar levels.even and hunger hormones completely balanced. Paleo guidelines for beginners:

Sounds simple, however going caveman successfully requires savvy:

SKIP ALL GRAINS

(whole grains and refined), dairy, packaged snacks, legumes and sugar in favor of vegetables, fruits, meats, eggs, seafood, nuts, fats, seeds and oils. For starters, you can follow these paleo diet principles.

PRECISE MOTIVATION

Most individuals turn to the Paleo diet to help with health issues such as gastrointestinal problems, allergies, and autoimmune diseases. Some need to feel good day-to-day or believe it is a healthy way to eat. Your main reason would help you determine the principles to follow and what you need to be careful about. Also, be strict about your guidelines for the very first month. It is a long enough time to start seeing good changes in your health.

CLEAN YOUR KITCHEN

Gather up all the "don't" foods listed on the Paleo diet, such as packaged foods, cereals, milk, cheese, vegetable oils, yogurt, and beans, you got it- and throw them in the trash. Doing all of this has one advantage: it's easy to avoid temptation when it's not there. But if you like to take baby steps at first, then it works just the same. You can probably cut out dairy during the first week, eliminate refined grains during the second week, and cut out grains during the third week, and so on until you're following the Paleo diet. In any case, make sure you buy whole foods; therefore, you have enough to that you can work with to create a Paleo diet meal plan.

FOLLOW THE 85/15 APPROACH

After the 1st 30 days, several experts suggest the 85/15 rule, which means that you stick strictly to the paleo diet 85% of the time and save 15% for non-paleo, whether that's one muesli bar (you could choose this from a paleo muesli recipe), one burger (bun and all) when cooking, or some smoothies. Focus on how you feel after introducing new things to the paleo diet. For example, if you have one scoop of delicious ice cream and wake up bloated the next day, you might decide that the future discomfort isn't worth it

COOK

Because the Paleo diet is based on fresh, whole foods, it's easier to prepare meals at home than at a restaurant, where it's hard to control what ingredients are there. So take advantage of this unique opportunity to experiment with new foods.

You may find it a bit challenging to buy a strange-looking vegetable at the market and ask the vendor for advice on how to prepare it perfectly. You can also search the internet or invest in a paleo diet cookbook for inspiration; that way, the meals will stay tasty and won't just be plain chicken breasts along with simple carrots and kale.

EXPECT 1 FAILURE (OR 2)

It's normal to slip into your usual eating habits when following the Paleo diet. However, you don't have to worry about failure. It's a good learning process. You can also seek out like-minded people who are already following this diet through local forums, groups, blogs, and Facebook and connect with them to take help and keep you on track - and keep you there.

LABEL DECODER

As you know, don't eat doughnuts, crackers and cookies, but a few foods are not paleo: nut butter jars; peanut butter (that's a legume); dried fruit along with added sugars; and lunchmeats, malt vinegar, soy sauce and other sauces and marinades (some consist of sugar, soy, preservatives and gluten). So when buying anything in a packet, make sure you check the list of all ingredients.

THINK ABOUT YOUR PLATE

We teach you to always reserve half your plate for vegetables, a quarter for lean protein, and the remaining quarter for whole grains. As you transition to a Paleo diet, stop saving room for grains. A balanced plate includes a palm-sized protein, one pan of fat, and veggies, veggies, veggies (fill the remaining container along with them).

REPLACE THE OIL

Instead of reaching for corn, canola or soybean oil for frying, you'll need to use lard or coconut oil. Really. Yes, it's good to cook with these good quality saturated fats because they are stable and don't oxidize when cooked (plus oxidation releases harmful free radicals). As for lard, animal fats - in this case from grass-fed cows - have been loaded with huge amounts of omega 3 and one form of fat known as conjugated linoleic acid, which some studies suggest may help you burn fat.

Some dietitians also recommend butter from grass-fed cows; however, many limit dairy products of all kinds. (The choice is yours.) For cold applications, you can use walnut oil, olive oil, and avocado oil.

EAT MEAT

Many people have limited meat in the Paleo diet because they believe it is harmful to health. You can eat meat too - just be sure it's good quality. So you can say goodbye to processed meats, which include salami, hot dogs and sausages.

Wild meats such as bison, boar and elk are excellent choices, followed by pasture-raised poultry as well as meat, and the last choice has to be grain-fed lean meats. And when it comes to seafood, choose wild-caught quite often, with low-mercury and sustainably sourced choices being best.

YOU CAN EASILY FOOL YOUR SWEET TOOTH.

Eliminating sugar is one of the primary difficult tasks for several people in the beginning. In the event that you like to indulge in a treat right after dinner, you can swap cookies or just for yourself for one piece of fruit. (For your sugar cravings, experts say the Paleo diet permits dried mango). Over time, your taste buds would adjust accordingly - and that Oreos you used to love so much may now become so sweet for you. Seriously, it can happen!

YOU CAN EAT OUT

On the paleo diet, it's possible to have a business dinner or brunch with your best friends. All you have to do is do a little digging for ingredients. First, you need to look at the menu beforehand and pick 1 or 2 options that you could paleo modify.

For example, it could be wild salmon and broccoli. (Also, ask for double the vegetables rather than rice pilaf.) Also, don't be shy about asking pertinent questions at the restaurant about what you're preparing and ask for adjustments if necessary.

EAT WHOLESOME, NUTRIENT-DENSE FOODS.If the food is not in the condition it was when it was pulled from the soil, then chances are it has been refined and is not optimal. By choosing foods straight from nature, we provide our bodies with the nutrients that are needed to heal our bodies.

AVOID NUTRIENT-POOR, PROCESSED AND REFINED FOODS THAT ARE PRODUCED IN FACTORIES

This means pasteurized dairy products, grains, seed oils (canola, cottonseed, corn, and soya), artificial sweeteners and refined sugar (high fructose corn syrup). Most of these foods rob the body of nutrients for digestion, which negates the primary goal of diet, which is to fuel the human body and provide it with nutrients for growth and repair. Yes, getting familiar with the paleo lifestyle would take some time. In the beginning, there may be some confusion as you work on changing your habits of grocery shopping, eating out and food preparation; therefore, it is essential to change it at a gradual pace that suits you perfectly. Additionally, know that most "non-paleo" foods need to be reworked to fit the paleo lifestyle.

FOOD FOR A HEALTHY DIGESTIVE SYSTEM

Gut and brain health is extremely important for overall health. To be successful, you need to focus on the signs your body is giving you. In case you find that eating dairy products causes certain digestive problems, then this is your body's way of telling you to avoid these foods! Keeping a food diary and food record could help you discover the latest trends and signs of food consumption. Digestive health is more important than many people think. Did you know that 60 to 80 percent of the immune system starts in the gut? If you were to constantly burden your digestion with certain irritating foods, then your immune system would be suppressed and your health would suffer greatly.

EAT FOODS THAT KEEP BLOOD SUGAR LEVELS STABLE

Have you ever felt weak or shaky between meals? Do you have fluctuations in your energy levels? Chances are your blood sugar levels rise and fall as a result of eating. If you eat sugar and white flour, then your blood sugar levels will spike and you will feel a rush of energy. While the body handles the sugar automatically, the blood sugar level also drops and you start feeling hungry and lethargic. Eating wholesome foods would provide the body with carbohydrates, enough protein and sufficient fats. This combination would allow blood sugar levels to rise even more slowly after meals and remain elevated between meals. Because the Paleo diet is all about eating whole foods, it could be suitable for everyone. The main thing is that it could easily be adapted to suit everyone. Keeping one journal of how you feel throughout the day could make the whole process go smoothly.

Author's note: This book has given you all the information you need to do this diet correctly and do it right. It is essential to understand what you are getting into when you embark on this diet, and this book gave you valuable information that you can use to your advantage and avoid the problems that can come with this diet. You want to stay healthy and make sure that your body can do what it needs to do. As with anything, we emphasize that if something seems wrong or unnatural, you will need to see a doctor to make sure you are safe and that your body can handle this diet. Use the knowledge in this book to get amazing recipes and learn directions for excellent meals for yourself. Consult your doctor before to starting new diet.

BREAKFAST RECIPES

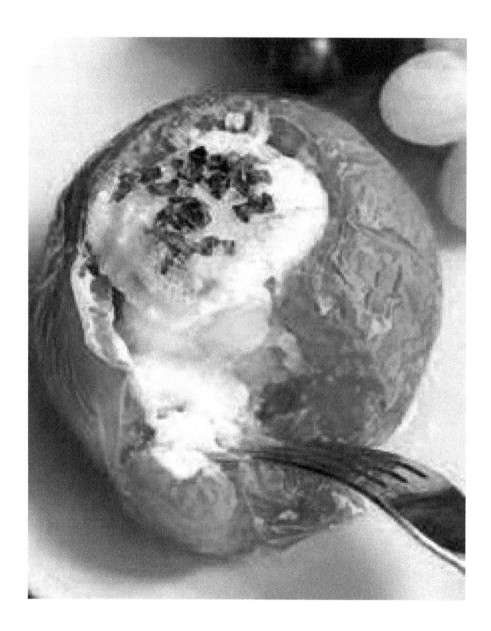

1) CHIA AND STRAWBERRY PORRIDGE

Preparation Time: 10 minutes   Cooking Time: 6 hours   Servings: 2

Ingredients:

- ✓ 2 tablespoons chia seeds
- ✓ ¼ cup water
- ✓ 1 green apple, cored and grated

Ingredients:

- ✓ 2 tablespoons coconut, desiccated 4 strawberries, halved
- ✓ ½ cup coconut milk
- ✓ 2 tablespoons hazelnuts

Directions:

- ❖ In your slow cooker, combine the chia seeds with water, apple, coconut strawberries, coconut milk and hazelnuts
- ❖ Stir, cover, cook on Low for 6 hours, divide into 2 bowls and serve for breakfast.

2) EASY PORRIDGE

Preparation Time: 10 minutes   Cooking Time: 6 hours   Servings: 3

Ingredients:

- ✓ 2 bananas, peeled and mashed
- ✓ ¾ cup almond meal 2 cups coconut milk
- ✓ 1 teaspoon cinnamon powder

Ingredients:

- ✓ ¼ cup flax meal
- ✓ ½ teaspoon ginger, grated A pinch of cloves, ground A pinch of nutmeg, ground

Directions:

- ❖ In your slow cooker, combine the bananas with the almond meal, coconut milk, cinnamon, flax meal, ginger, cloves and nutmeg
- ❖ Toss, cover, cook on Low for 6 hours, divide into bowls and serve.

3) CHIA SEEDS PORRIDGE

Preparation Time: 10 minutes   Cooking Time: 7 hours   Servings: 3

Ingredients:

- ✓ 1 and ½ cups almond milk 2 tablespoons flaxseed
- ✓ 3 tablespoons chia seeds
- ✓ 3 tablespoons coconut, shredded and unsweetened A handful almonds, chopped

Ingredients:

- ✓ 1 teaspoon vanilla extract 1 tablespoon gelatin
- ✓ 1 mango, peeled and cubed

Directions:

- ❖ In your slow cooker, combine the milk with flaxseed, chia seeds, coconut, almonds, vanilla and gelatin
- ❖ Toss, cover and cook on Low for 7 hours.
- ❖ Divide into bowls, sprinkle mango pieces on top and serve.

4) TASTY VEGGIE FRITTATA

Preparation Time: 10 minutes   Cooking Time: 2 hours   Servings: 4

Ingredients:

- ✓ Cooking spray 6 eggs
- ✓ 4 ounces mushrooms, chopped 1 teaspoon garlic powder
- ✓ A pinch of black pepper

Ingredients:

- ✓ ¼ cup spinach, chopped 2 green onions, chopped
- ✓ ¼ cup cherry tomatoes, chopped 1 teaspoon olive oil

Directions:

- ❖ Spray your slow cooker with cooking spray and leave aside for now.
- ❖ Heat up a pan with the oil over medium heat; add onions, spinach, mushrooms and tomatoes
- ❖ Stir and sauté for a couple of minutes.

- ❖ Transfer this to your slow cooker, add eggs, a pinch of pepper and garlic powder, stir gently
- ❖ Cover and cook on High for 2 hours.
- ❖ Divide between plates and serve hot

5) EGGS IN PEPPER RINGS

Preparation Time: 10 minutes   Cooking Time: 10   minutes   Servings: 4

Ingredients:

- ✓ 1 big sweet pepper
- ✓ 4 eggs
- ✓ ½ teaspoon ground paprika

Ingredients:

- ✓ ¼ teaspoon ground black pepper
- ✓ Cooking spray

Directions:

- ❖ Remove the seeds from the sweet pepper and slice it on 4 rings.
- ❖ Then preheat the skillet well and put the pepper rings in it.
- ❖ Cook the pepper rings for 1 minute from each side over the medium heat.

- ❖ Then spray the vegetables with cooking spray and crack the eggs inside every pepper ring.
- ❖ Sprinkle the meal with ground paprika and ground black pepper.
- ❖ Cook it for 5 minutes over the medium heat.

6) NUTRITIOUS BREAKFAST HASHES

Preparation Time: 15 minutes   Cooking Time: 10   minutes   Servings: 3

Ingredients:

- ✓ 1 sweet potato, peeled
- ✓ 1 tablespoon olive oil
- ✓ 1 zucchini, grated
- ✓ ½ teaspoon salt

Ingredients:

- ✓ 1 egg, beaten
- ✓ 1 teaspoon chili flakes
- ✓ 2 tablespoons coconut flour

Directions:

- ❖ Grate the sweet potato and put it in the bowl.
- ❖ Add grated zucchini, salt, egg, chili flakes, and coconut flour.
- ❖ Stir the vegetable mixture until homogenous.
- ❖ Then heat up the skillet.

- ❖ Pour the olive oil inside.
- ❖ Make the medium size hashes with the help of 2 spoons
- ❖ Put them in the hot skillet.
- ❖ Cook the hashes for 4 minutes from each side over the medium heat.

7) STUFFED TOMATOES WITH EGGS

Preparation Time: 15 minutes   Cooking Time: 10 minutes   Servings: 2

Ingredients:

- ✓ 2 medium tomatoes
- ✓ 2 eggs
- ✓ 1 teaspoon dried oregano

Ingredients:

- ✓ ½ teaspoon dried parsley
- ✓ 1 teaspoon olive oil

Directions:

- ❖ Cut the one end of the tomatoes and remove all tomato meat with the help of the scooper.
- ❖ Then sprinkle the tomatoes with dried oregano and parsley.
- ❖ After this, crack the eggs inside the tomatoes.
- ❖ Brush the vegetables with olive oil gently.

- ❖ Preheat the oven to 365F.
- ❖ Put the stuffed tomatoes on the tray and transfer it in the oven.
- ❖ Cook the meal for 10 minutes or until the eggs are firm

8)   EGG CUPS

Preparation Time: 15   minutes   Cooking Time: 12   minutes   Servings: 4

Ingredients:

- ✓ 4 eggs, beaten
- ✓ 1 tablespoon coconut flour
- ✓ 4 bacon slices

Ingredients:

- ✓ ½ teaspoon salt
- ✓ 1 teaspoon sesame oil
- ✓ ½ teaspoon chili powder

Directions:

- ❖ Brush the muffin molds with sesame oil.
- ❖ Then put the bacon in the muffin molds in the shape of the wholes.
- ❖ In the mixing bowl mix up beaten eggs, coconut flour, salt, and chili powder.

- ❖ Pour the egg mixture in the bacon wholes.
- ❖ Preheat the oven to 360F.
- ❖ Put the molds with a meal in the oven and cook for 12 minutes.

9)   HEARTY BREAKFAST PORK MIX

Preparation Time: 10 minutes   Cooking Time: 8 hours   Servings: 4

Ingredients:

- ✓ 1 medium pork butt
- ✓ 1 teaspoon coriander, ground
- ✓ 1 tablespoon oregano, dried
- ✓ 1 tablespoon cumin powder
- ✓ 2 tablespoons chili powder

Ingredients:

- ✓ 2 onions, chopped
- ✓ A pinch of black pepper
- ✓ 1 teaspoon lime juice
- ✓ 4 eggs, already fried
- ✓ 2 avocados, peeled, pitted and sliced

Directions:

- ❖ In a bowl, mix pork butt with coriander, oregano, cumin, chili powder, onions and a pinch of black pepper, rub well
- ❖ Transfer to your slow cooker and cook on Low for 8 hours.

- ❖ Shred meat, divide between plates and serve with fried eggs and avocado slices on top and with lime juice all over.

10) DELICIOUS SAUSAGE AND EGGS CASSEROLE

Preparation Time: 10 minutes   Cooking Time: 5 hours   Servings: 6

Ingredients:

- ✓ 1 broccoli head, florets separated
- ✓ 10 eggs, whisked
- ✓ 12 ounces sausages, cooked and sliced

Ingredients:

- ✓ 2 garlic cloves, minced
- ✓ A pinch of sea salt Cooking spray
- ✓ Black pepper to the taste

Directions:

- ❖ Spray your slow cooker with the cooking spray and layer half of the broccoli florets.
- ❖ Add a layer of sausages, and then add half of the whisked eggs, a pinch of salt and some black pepper.
- ❖ Add garlic, the rest of the broccoli, sausages and the rest of the eggs.
- ❖ Cover and cook on Low for 5 hours.
- ❖ Leave casserole to cool down, slice, divide between plates and serve.

11) SPICED ORANGE BREAKFAST COUSCOUS

Preparation Time: 5   minutes   Cooking Time: 15   minutes   Servings: 4

Ingredients:

- ✓ 3 cups orange juice
- ✓ 1.1/2 cups couscous
- ✓ 1 teaspoon ground cinnamon
- ✓ 1/4 teaspoon ground cloves

Ingredients:

- ✓ 1/2 cup dried fruit
- ✓ 1/2 cup chopped almonds

Directions:

- ❖ Take the orange juice to a boil. Add the couscous, cinnamon, and cloves and remove from heat
- ❖ Shield the pan and allow sitting until the couscous softens.
- ❖ Fluff the couscous and stir in the dried fruit and nuts
- ❖ Serve - immediately. Pecans and syrup. Serve hot.

12) BROILED GRAPEFRUIT WITH CINNAMON PITAS

Preparation Time: 5   minutes   Cooking Time: 15   minutes   Servings: 4

Ingredients:

- ✓ 2 whole-wheat pitas cut into wedges

Ingredients:

- ✓ 2 tablespoons coconut oil, melted

Directions:

- ❖ Preheat the oven to 375°F. Line a baking sheet with parchment paper.
- ❖ Spread pita wedges in a single layer on a baking sheet and brush with melted coconut oil.
- ❖ In a small bowl, combine the cinnamon and brown sugar and sprinkle over the pita wedges.
- ❖ Bake in preheated oven until the wedges are crisp, about 8 minutes
- ❖ Transfer the pita wedges to a plate and set aside.
- ❖ Turn the oven to broil. Drip the maple syrup over the top of the grapefruit, if using
- ❖ Broil until the syrup bubbles and begins to crystallize, 3 to 5 minutes. Serve immediately

13) BREAKFAST PARFAITS

Cooking Time: 15 minutes   Servings: 4

Ingredients:

- ✓ One 14-ounce cans coconut milk, refrigerated overnight
- ✓ 1 cup granola

Ingredients:

- ✓ 1/2 cup walnuts
- ✓ 1 cup sliced strawberries or other seasonal berries

Directions:

- ❖ Pour off the canned coconut-milk liquid and retain the solids.
- ❖ In two parfait glasses, layer the coconut-milk solids, granola, walnuts, and strawberries.
- ❖ Serve immediately

14) BARLEY BREAKFAST BOWL

Preparation Time: 5 minutes   Cooking Time: 15 minutes   Servings: 4

Ingredients:

- ✓ 1.1/2 cups pearl barley
- ✓ 3.3/4 cups water
- ✓ Large pinch salt

Ingredients:

- ✓ 1.1/2 cups dried cranberries
- ✓ 3 cups sweetened vanilla plant-based milk
- ✓ 2 tablespoons slivered almonds (optional)

Directions:

- ❖ Put the barley, water, and salt. Bring to a boil.
- ❖ Divide the barley into 6 jars or single-serving storage containers. Attached the 1/4 cup of dried cranberries to each
- ❖ Pour 1/2 cup of plant-based milk into each. Attached the 1 teaspoon of slivered almonds (if using) to each
- ❖ Close the jars tightly with lids.

15) ORANGE FRENCH TOAST

Preparation Time: 5 minutes   Cooking Time: 15 minutes   Servings: 4

Ingredients:

- ✓ 3 very ripe bananas
- ✓ 1 cup unsweetened nondairy milk
- ✓ Zest and juice of 1 orange
- ✓ 1 teaspoon ground cinnamon

Ingredients:

- ✓ 1/4 teaspoon grated nutmeg
- ✓ 4 slices French bread
- ✓ tablespoon coconut oil

Directions:

- ❖ Blend the bananas, almond milk, orange juice and zest, cinnamon, and nutmeg and blend until smooth
- ❖ Dip the bread in the mixture for 5 minutes on each side.
- ❖ While the bread soaks, heat a griddle or sauté pan over medium- high heat. Melt the coconut oil in the pan and swirl to coat
- ❖ Cook the bread slices until golden brown on both sides, about 5 minutes each. Serve immediately

16) PUMPKIN PANCAKES

Preparation Time: 5 minutes   Cooking Time: 15 minutes   Servings: 4

Ingredients:

- ✓ cups unsweetened almond milk
- ✓ 1 teaspoon apple cider vinegar
- ✓ 2.1/2 cups whole-wheat flour
- ✓ 2 tablespoons baking powder
- ✓ 1/2 teaspoon baking soda

Ingredients:

- ✓ 1 teaspoon sea salt
- ✓ 1 teaspoon pumpkin pie
- ✓ 1/2 cup canned pumpkin purée 1 cup water
- ✓ 1 tablespoon coconut oil

Directions:

- ❖ Dip together the flour, baking powder, baking soda, salt and pumpkin pie spice.
- ❖ In another large bowl, combine the almond milk mixture, pumpkin
- ❖ purée, and water, whisking to mix well.
- ❖ Add the wet ingredients to the dry ingredients and fold together until the dry ingredients are just moistened
- ❖ You will still have a few streaks of flour in the bowl.

- ❖ In a nonstick pan or griddle over medium-high heat, melt the coconut oil and swirl to coat
- ❖ Pour the batter into the pan 1/4 cup at a time and cook until the pancakes are browned, about 5 minutes per side
- ❖ Serve immediately

17) VANILLA PANCAKES

Preparation Time: 10 minutes   Cooking Time: 15 minutes   Servings: 6

Ingredients:

- • ½ cup of coconut milk
- • 2 eggs, beaten
- • 1 teaspoon vanilla extract
- • 1 teaspoon baking powder

Ingredients:

- • 1 teaspoon lemon juice
- • 1 cup almond flour
- • 1 tablespoon raw honey

Directions:

- ❖ In the big bowl mix up coconut milk and eggs.
- ❖ Add vanilla extract, baking powder, and lemon juicer.
- ❖ When the liquid is homogenous, add the almond flour.
- ❖ Stir the mixture with the help of the hand whisker until it is homogenous and without lumps.
- ❖ Preheat the non-stick skillet well.

- ❖ Then pour the pancake batter in the hot skillet with the help of the ladle (1 ladle = 1 pancake).
- ❖ Cook the pancake for 1 minute and flip it on another side
- ❖ Cook it for 30 seconds more or until the pancake is light brown.
- ❖ Repeat the same steps with all remaining batter.
- ❖ Sprinkle the cooker pancakes with honey.

18) APPLE BUTTER

Preparation Time: 10 minutes   Cooking Time: 8 hours   Servings: 10

Ingredients:

- Juice of 1 lemon
- 1 teaspoon allspice
- 1 teaspoon clove, ground 1 teaspoon ginger powder

Ingredients:

- 3 pounds apples, peeled, cored and chopped 1 tablespoon cinnamon, ground
- 1 and ½ cups water
- ¼ teaspoon nutmeg, ground 1 cup maple syrup

Directions:

- ❖ In your slow cooker, mix apples with water, lemon juice
- ❖ Then allspice, clove, ginger powder, cinnamon, maple syrup and nutmeg.
- ❖ Stir, cover and cook on Low for 8 hours.

- ❖ Leave your mix to cool down for 10 minutes, blend using an immersion blender and pour into small jars.
- ❖ Serve for breakfast!

19) DELICIOUS BREAKFAST BOWLS

Preparation Time: 10 minutes   Cooking Time: 8 hours   Servings: 4

Ingredients:

- ½ cup almonds, soaked for 12 hours and drained
- ½ cup walnuts, soaked for 12 hours and drained 2 apples, peeled, cored and cubed
- 1 butternut squash, peeled and cubed 1 teaspoon cinnamon powder

Ingredients:

- 1 tablespoon coconut sugar
- ½ teaspoon nutmeg, ground 1 cup coconut milk
- Maple syrup for serving

Directions:

- ❖ Put almonds and walnuts in your blender, add some of the soaking water, blend really well and transfer to your slow cooker.
- ❖ Add apples, squash, cinnamon, coconut sugar, nutmeg and coconut milk

- ❖ Stir, cover and cook on Low for 8 hours.
- ❖ Use a potato masher to mash the whole mix, divide into bowls and serve.

20) BREAKFAST BURGER WITH EGGS

Preparation Time: 10 minutes   Cooking Time: 15 minutes   Servings: 2

Ingredients:

- 2 eggs
- 8 oz ground beef
- ½ teaspoon dried parsley
- ½ teaspoon salt

Ingredients:

- ½ teaspoon ground black pepper
- ½ teaspoon dried garlic
- 1 teaspoon olive oil

Directions:

- ❖ In the mixing bowl mix up ground beef, parsley, salt, ground black pepper, and dried garlic.
- ❖ When the mixture is homogenous, make 2 balls (burgers).
- ❖ Preheat the skillet over the medium heat until it is hot and pour the olive oil inside.
- ❖ Place the burgers in the oil and cook them for 3 minutes from each side over the medium heat.

- ❖ Then transfer the burgers on the serving plates.
- ❖ Clean the skillet and crack the eggs inside.
- ❖ Cook them for 4 minutes or until the eggs are firm.
- ❖ Put the cooked eggs over the burgers

21) VEGETABLE HASH WITH BACON

Cooking Time: 10 minutes   Servings: 2

Ingredients:

- 3 oz bacon, chopped
- 1 yellow onion, chopped
- 1 tablespoon sunflower oil

Ingredients:

- ½ teaspoon ground black pepper
- ½ teaspoon salt
- 1 sweet pepper, chopped

Directions:

- ❖ Preheat the skillet well and put the bacon inside.
- ❖ Cook it for 2 minutes over the medium heat.
- ❖ Then add chopped onion and sprinkle with ground black pepper and salt.
- ❖ Mix up the mixture and cook it for 3 minutes more.
- ❖ Add the sunflower oil and chopped sweet pepper. Mix up the hash well.
- ❖ Close the lid and cook the meal for 5 minutes over the medium-low heat.

22) BACON AND LEEKS BREAKFAST CASSEROLE

Preparation Time: 10 minutes   Cooking Time: 2 hours   Servings: 8

Ingredients:

- 2 leeks, sliced
- 5 bacon slices, cooked and chopped A pinch of salt and black pepper
- 6 eggs, whisked
- 2 teaspoons thyme, chopped 2 cups coconut cream

Ingredients:

- 1 cup coconut milk
- 1 tablespoon mustard
- A pinch of nutmeg, ground
- ½ cup parsley, chopped Cooking spray

Directions:

- ❖ In a bowl, combine the eggs with thyme, salt, pepper coconut cream
- ❖ Then milk, mustard, nutmeg and parsley and whisk well.
- ❖ Grease your slow cooker with cooking spray
- ❖ Arrange bacon and leeks on the bottom, pour the eggs mix, spread, cover and cook on High for 2 hours.
- ❖ 3.Slice, divide between plates and serve for breakfast

23) STRAWBERRIES BREAKFAST MIX

Cooking Time: 8 minutes   Servings: 8

Ingredients:

- 2 cups strawberries
- 2 cups almond milk 6 cups water

Ingredients:

- 1 cup coconut flakes
- 1 teaspoon cinnamon powder
- 1 teaspoon vanilla extract

Directions:

- ❖ In your slow cooker, combine the strawberries with almond milk, water, coconut, cinnamon and vanilla
- ❖ Toss, cover and cook on Low for 8 hours.
- ❖ Divide into bowls and serve.

24) CINNAMON AND RAISINS OATMEAL

Preparation Time: 10 minutes   Cooking Time: 8 hours   Servings: 2

Ingredients:

- ¼ cup walnuts, chopped
- 1 tablespoon coconut flour 1 tablespoon flax meal
- 1 cup cashew milk

Ingredients:

- ¼ teaspoon cinnamon powder 1 teaspoon chia seeds
- 2 tablespoons raisins
- 1 tablespoon stevia

Directions:

- ❖ In your slow cooker, combine the walnuts with coconut flour, flax meal, cashew milk
- ❖ Then cinnamon, chia seeds, raisins and stevia, toss, cover and cook on Low for 8 hours.

- ❖ Divide into bowls and serve.

25) PROTEIN SMOOTHIE

Preparation Time: 5 minutes   Cooking Time: 4   minutes   Servings: 1

Ingredients:

- 2 oz blueberries, frozen
- 2 oz strawberries, frozen
- 1 teaspoon collagen hydrolysate

Ingredients:

- ½ cup of coconut milk
- 1 teaspoon raw honey
- ❖

Directions:

- ❖ Put the frozen blueberries and strawberries in the blender.
- ❖ Add collagen hydrolysate and coconut milk.
- ❖ Blend the mixture until it is smooth

- ❖
- ❖ Sprinkle the eggs with Italian seasonings mixture and close the
- ❖ lid.
- ❖ Cook the eggs over the medium heat for 5 minutes.

26) HERBED FRIED EGGS

Preparation Time: 10 minutes   Cooking Time: 5   minutes   Servings: 4

Ingredients:

- 4 eggs
- 1 teaspoon Italian seasonings
- 1 teaspoon dried thyme

Ingredients:

- ¼ teaspoon salt
- 2 tablespoons sunflower oil

Directions:

- ❖ In the mixing bowl mix up Italians seasonings, dried thyme, and salt.
- ❖ Heat up the skillet until it is hot.
- ❖ Add the sunflower oil and crack the eggs.

- ❖ Sprinkle the eggs with Italian seasonings mixture and close the lid.
- ❖ Cook the eggs over the medium heat for 5 minutes.

27) BANANA PANCAKES

Preparation Time: 15 minutes   Cooking Time: 15 minutes   Servings: 6

Ingredients:

- 3 bananas, peeled
- 3 eggs, beaten
- 1 cup almond flour
- ½ teaspoon baking soda
- 1 teaspoon lemon juice

Ingredients:

- 1 teaspoon lemon zest, grated
- 1 teaspoon ground cinnamon
- ¼ cup of coconut milk
- ¼ cup yacon syrup

Directions:

- ❖ Chop the bananas roughly and put in the blender.
- ❖ Add eggs, almond flour, baking soda
- ❖ Then lemon juice, lemon zest, ground cinnamon, and coconut milk.
- ❖ Blend the mixture until you get a smooth batter
- ❖ It will take approximately 5-7 minutes.
- ❖ Preheat the non-stick skillet well.

- ❖ With the help of the ladle make the pancake in the skillet
- ❖ Cook it for 1 minute from each side
- ❖ The cooked pancake should have a light brown color.
- ❖ Repeat the same steps with the remaining pancake batter.
- ❖ Sprinkle the cooked pancakes with yacon syrup.

28) PEAR BREAKFAST MIX

Preparation Time: 10 minutes   Cooking Time: 8 hours   Servings: 4

Ingredients:

- 6 pears, cored, peeled and chopped
- 2 tablespoons coconut oil, melted
- 6 ounces coconut milk
- 2/3 cup coconut butter
-

Ingredients:

- 1 tablespoon vanilla extract
- 3 cups coconut, shredded
- ½ teaspoon cinnamon powder

Directions:

- ❖ In your slow cooker, combine the pears with the coconut oil, milk, coconut butter, vanilla, coconut and cinnamon

- ❖ Toss, cover and cook on Low for 8 hours.
- ❖ Divide into bowls and serve for breakfast.

29) CHICKEN FRITTATA

Preparation Time: 15 minutes   Cooking Time: 20 minutes   Servings: 5

Ingredients:

- 5 eggs, beaten
- 4 oz chicken fillet
- 1 teaspoon chili flakes
- 1 teaspoon salt
- 1 teaspoon dried dill

Ingredients:

- 1 teaspoon ground black pepper
- 1 tomato, chopped
- 1 tablespoon olive oil
- 1 teaspoon coconut oil

Directions:

- ❖ Grind the chicken and mix it up with chili flakes, salt, dried dill, ground black pepper, and olive oil.
- ❖ Put the mixture in the skillet and cook it for 10 minutes over the medium heat
- ❖ Stir it from time to time to avoid burning.

- ❖ Then add coconut oil and stir the mixture until coconut oil is melted.
- ❖ After this, add beaten eggs and stir the ingredients.
- ❖ Close the lid and cook the frittata for 10 minutes

30) BUTTERNUT SQUASH BOWLS

Preparation Time: 10 minutes   Cooking Time: 6 hours   Servings: 3

Ingredients:

- 1 banana, peeled and chopped
- 1 teaspoon cinnamon powder
- 1 cup coconut, shredded

Ingredients:

- ½ cup butternut squash puree
- ½ cup coconut milk

Directions:

- ❖ In your slow cooker, combine the banana with the cinnamon, coconut, squash puree and coconut milk
- ❖ Toss, cover and cook on Low for 6 hours.

- ❖ Divide into bowls and serve for breakfast

31) COCONUT CREPES

Preparation Time: 10 minutes   Cooking Time: 10 minutes   Servings: 6

Ingredients:

- 1 cup coconut flour
- 2 tablespoons coconut flakes
- 1 teaspoon vanilla extract
- 3 eggs, beaten
- ¼ cup Erythritol

Ingredients:

- ¼ teaspoon ground cardamom
- ½ teaspoon baking soda
- 1 teaspoon apple cider vinegar
- 1/3 cup coconut milk

Directions:

- ❖ Put all ingredients from the list above in the big bowl and mix up until you get the smooth batter.
- ❖ After this, preheat the non-sticky skillet well.
- ❖ Pour the crepe batter in the preheated
- ❖ Skillet with the help of the ladle and flatten the batter in the shape of the crepe.

- ❖ Cook it for 1 minute.
- ❖ Carefully flip the crepe on another side and cook it for 30 seconds more.
- ❖ Repeat the same steps with the remaining batter

32) PORTOBELLO BACON SANDWICH

Preparation Time: 10 minutes   Cooking Time: 6 minutes   Servings: 4

Ingredients:

- 8 Portobello mushroom caps
- 8 bacon slices
- 1 teaspoon olive oil
- 1 teaspoon sunflower oil

Ingredients:

- 1 teaspoon dried rosemary
- 1 teaspoon salt
- 1 teaspoon dried thyme

Directions:

- ❖ Preheat the grill to 375F.
- ❖ Sprinkle the mushroom caps with salt, dried rosemary, and thyme.
- ❖ Then put them in the preheated grill.

- ❖ Place the bacon in the grill too.
- ❖ Sprinkle the mushrooms and bacon with olive oil and cook them for 3 minutes from each side.
- ❖ Then put the bacon on 2 mushroom caps, sprinkle with sunflower oil and cover with remaining mushroom caps

33) CHIA PUDDING

Preparation Time: 3 hours   Cooking Time: 10   minutes   Servings: 3

Ingredients:

- 4 tablespoons chia seeds
- 1 teaspoon tapioca starch/flour
- 1 teaspoon vanilla extract

Ingredients:

- 1 ½ cup of coconut milk
- 2 teaspoons raw honey
- 1 teaspoon coconut flakes

Directions:

- ❖ In the mixing bowl mix up chia seeds, tapioca starch, vanilla extract, coconut milk, and coconut flakes.
- ❖ Add raw honey and stir the mixture until homogenous.
- ❖ Then pour the pudding in the serving jars and leave for 3 hours in the fridge.

34) TOMATO AND KALE SCRAMBLE

Preparation Time: 10 minutes   Cooking Time: 10   minutes   Servings: 1

Ingredients:

- 2 eggs, whisked
- ¼ teaspoon rosemary, dried
- ½ cup cherry tomatoes halved 1 and ½ cups kale, chopped

Ingredients:

- ½ teaspoon coconut oil, melted 3 tablespoons water
- 1 teaspoon balsamic vinegar
- ¼ avocado, peeled, pitted and chopped

Directions:

- ❖ Heat up a pan with the oil over medium heat, add the water, kale, rosemary, and tomatoes, stir, cover and cook for 5 minutes.
- ❖ Add the eggs, stir and scramble everything for 4 minutes more.
- ❖ Add the vinegar, toss, transfer this to a plate, top with chopped avocado and serve.

35) BREAKFAST STUFFED SWEET POTATO

Preparation Time: 15 minutes   Cooking Time: 25   minutes   Servings: 2

Ingredients:

- 2 sweet potatoes
- 2 teaspoons coconut oil, softened
- 1 teaspoon salt
- ½ teaspoon chili powder

Ingredients:

- ½ teaspoon dried garlic
- 1 tablespoon chives, chopped
- 4 oz ground beef

Directions:

- ❖ Preheat the oven to 365F.
- ❖ Wrap the sweet potatoes in the foil and put it in the oven. Cook the vegetables for 15 minutes.
- ❖ Then discard the foil and make the horizontal cut on every sweet potato.
- ❖ Mash the sweet potato pulp gently with the help of the fork.
- ❖ Then in the mixing bowl mix up salt, chili powder, garlic, and chives.
- ❖ Toss the coconut oil in the skillet.
- ❖ Add ground beef and cook it for 3 minutes.
- ❖ Mix up the meat and add chili powder mixture.
- ❖ Cook the ground beef for 7 minutes more.
- ❖ Then fill the sweet potatoes with the ground beef mixture.

36) BREAKFAST CARNITAS

Preparation Time: 15 minutes   Cooking Time: 65 minutes   Servings: 4

Ingredients:

- 8 oz pork shoulder, boneless
- 1 white onion, peeled
- 1 chili pepper
- 1 cup beef broth
- 1 teaspoon salt

Ingredients:

- 1 teaspoon peppercorn
- 1 garlic clove, peeled
- 1 teaspoon ground black pepper
- 1 teaspoon lemon juice
- 1 teaspoon fresh parsley, chopped

Directions:

- ❖ Chop the pork shoulder roughly and put it in the pan.
- ❖ Add onion, chili pepper, beef broth, salt, peppercorn, garlic clove, ground black pepper, and close the lid.
- ❖ Cook the meat mixture over the medium heat for 65 minutes.
- ❖ Then remove the meat from the liquid and shred it with the help of the fork.
- ❖ Sprinkle the shredded meat with lemon juice and parsley
- ❖

37) SWEET POTATO AND KALE HASH

Preparation Time: 10 minutes   Cooking Time: 15 minutes   Servings: 2

Ingredients:

- ✓ 1 sweet potato
- ✓ 2 tablespoons olive oil
- ✓ 1/2 onion, chopped
- ✓ 1 carrot, peeled and chopped
- ✓ 2 garlic cloves, minced

Ingredients:

- ✓ 1/2 teaspoon dried thyme
- ✓ 1 cup chopped kale
- ✓ Sea salt
- ✓ Freshly ground black pepper

Directions:

- ❖ Pierce the sweet potato and microwave on high until soft, about 5 minutes
- ❖ Remove from the microwave and cut into 1/4-inch cubes.
- ❖ In a large nonstick sauté pan, heat the olive oil over medium-high heat. Add the onion and carrot
- ❖ Cook until softened, about 5 minutes. Attach the garlic and thyme until the garlic is fragrant, about 30 seconds.
- ❖ Add the sweet potatoes and cook until the potatoes begin to brown, about 7 minutes
- ❖ Then the kale and cook just until it wilts, 1 to 2 minutes
- ❖ Season with salt and pepper. Serve immediately.

38) SAVORY OATMEAL PORRIDGE

Preparation Time: 5 minutes   Cooking Time: 20 minutes   Servings: 4

Ingredients:

- ✓ 2 1/2 cups vegetable broth
- ✓ 2 1/2 cups milk
- ✓ 1/2 cup steel-cut oats
- ✓ 1 tablespoon faro

Ingredients:

- ✓ ½ cup slivered almonds
- ✓ 1/4 cup nutritional yeast
- ✓ 2 cups old-fashioned rolled oats
- ✓ 1/2 teaspoon salt (optional)

Directions:

- ❖ Take the broth and almond milk to a boil. Add the oats, faro, almond slivers, and nutritional yeast
- ❖ Cook over medium-high heat for 20 minutes, stirring occasionally.
- ❖ Add the rolled oats and cook for another 5 minutes, until creamy. Stir in the salt (if using).
- ❖ Divide into 4 single-serving containers. Let cool before sealing the lids.

39) PUMPKIN STEEL-CUT OATS

Preparation Time: 15 minutes Cooking Time: 25 minutes Servings: 4

Ingredients:

- ✓ 3 cups water
- ✓ 1 cup steel-cut oats
- ✓ 1/2 cup canned pumpkin purée

Ingredients:

- ✓ 1/4 cup pumpkin seeds (pipits)
- ✓ 2 tablespoons maple syrup Pinch salt

Directions:

- ❖ Whip and reduce the heat to low.
- ❖ Simmer until the oats are soft, 20 to 30 minutes, continuing to stir occasionally.
- ❖ Stir in the pumpkin purée and continue cooking on low for 3 to 5 minutes longer

- ❖ Blend in the pumpkin seeds and maple syrup, and season with the salt.
- ❖ Divide the oatmeal into 4 single-serving containers. Let cool before sealing the lids

40) CINNAMON AND SPICE OVERNIGHT OATS

Preparation Time: 15 minutes Cooking Time: 20 minutes Servings: 3

Ingredients:

- ✓ 2.1/2 cups old-fashioned rolled oats
- ✓ 5 tablespoons pumpkin seeds (pipits)
- ✓ 5 tablespoons chopped pecans
- ✓ 5 cups unsweetened plant-based milk

Ingredients:

- ✓ 21/2 teaspoons maple syrup or agave syrup
- ✓ 1/2 to 1 teaspoon salt
- ✓ 1/2 to 1 teaspoon ground cinnamon
- ✓ 1/2 to 1 teaspoon ground ginger

Directions:

- ❖ Line up 5 wide-mouth pint jars. In each jar, combine 1/2 cup of oats, 1 tablespoon of pumpkin seeds, 1 tablespoon of pecans
- ❖ Then 1 cup of plant-based milk, 1/2 teaspoon of maple syrup, 1 pinch of salt, 1 pinch of cinnamon, and 1 pinch of ginger.

- ❖ Stir the ingredients in each jar. Close the jars tightly with lids. To serve, top with fresh fruit (if using)

LUNCH RECIPES

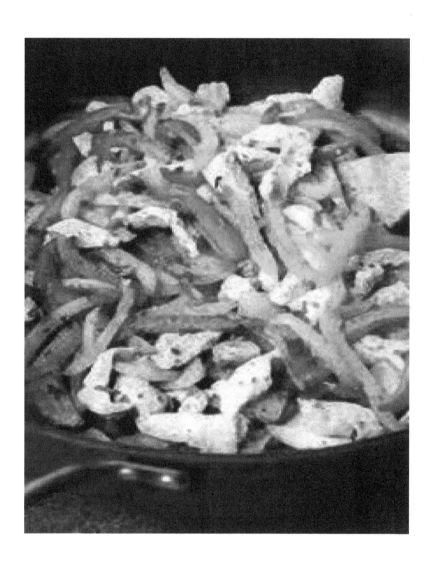

41) JALAPENO CHILI

Preparation Time: 10 minutes　　　Cooking Time: 40 minutes　　　Servings: 4

Ingredients:

- ✓ 8 oz ground beef
- ✓ 2 jalapeno pepper, sliced
- ✓ 3 oz bacon, chopped
- ✓ ½ cup tomatoes, diced
- ✓ 1 tablespoon tomato paste
- ✓ 1 cup of water
- ✓ 1 sweet pepper, chopped

Ingredients:

- ✓ ½ teaspoon ground cumin
- ✓ ½ teaspoon dried thyme
- ✓ ½ teaspoon ground paprika
- ✓ 1 teaspoon salt
- ✓ 1 onion, diced
- ✓ 1 teaspoon coconut oil

Directions:

- ❖ Put the coconut oil in the pan and melt it.
- ❖ Add ground beef, ground cumin, thyme, paprika, and salt.
- ❖ Mix up well and add diced onion.
- ❖ Close the lid and cook the beef mixture for 10 minutes over the medium-low heat.
- ❖ Preheat the skillet until it is hot and put the chopped bacon inside.
- ❖ Cook it until golden brown.
- ❖ Then add the bacon in the ground beef mixture.
- ❖ Add diced tomatoes, jalapeno pepper, sweet pepper, and water.
- ❖ After this, add tomato paste and stir the mixture until it will turn into a red color.
- ❖ Close the lid and simmer the chili over the medium heat for 25 minutes.

42) CAULIFLOWER WITH CHICKEN FAJITA

Preparation Time: 10 minutes　　　Cooking Time: 20 minutes　　　Servings: 4

Ingredients:

- ✓ 1 cup cauliflower, chopped
- ✓ 12 oz chicken fillet
- ✓ 1 teaspoon taco seasonings
- ✓ 1 red onion, sliced
- ✓ 1 teaspoon ground turmeric

Ingredients:

- ✓ 1 tablespoon coconut cream
- ✓ ½ teaspoon salt
- ✓ 1 teaspoon fresh cilantro, chopped
- ✓ 1 teaspoon coconut oil

Directions:

- ❖ Cut the chicken fillet on the strips and sprinkle with taco seasonings, ground turmeric, and salt.
- ❖ Then put the coconut oil in the skillet and melt it.
- ❖ Put the chicken strips in the hot skillet in one layer and cook for 4 minutes from each side over the medium heat.
- ❖ Then add red onion and mix up well. Add cauliflower, coconut cream, and fresh cilantro.
- ❖ Carefully mix up the mixture and close the lid.
- ❖ Preheat the oven to 365F.
- ❖ Put the skillet with a meal in the preheated oven and cook for 10 minutes.

43) TOMATO MEATBALLS

Preparation Time: 20 minutes   Cooking Time: 25 minutes   Servings: 5

Ingredients:

- ✓ 1 cup ground chicken
- ✓ 10 oz ground pork
- ✓ ½ zucchini, grated
- ✓ 1 teaspoon chili flakes
- ✓ 1 teaspoon Italian seasonings
- ✓ ½ teaspoon ground black pepper

Ingredients:

- ✓ 1 teaspoon ground nutmeg
- ✓ 1 tablespoon tapioca flour
- ✓ ½ cup crushed tomatoes
- ✓ 1 teaspoon coconut cream
- ✓ 1 teaspoon coconut oil

Directions:

- ❖ Make the meatballs: in the mixing bowl mix up ground chicken, grated zucchini, ground pork, chili flakes, and Italian seasonings.
- ❖ Then add ground black pepper and ground nutmeg. Mix up the meat mixture until it is smooth and make the small meatballs.
- ❖ After this, grease the baking tray with coconut oil and put the meatballs in it in one layer.
- ❖ Preheat the oven to 365F.
- ❖ Put the tray with meatballs in the oven and bake them for 10 minutes.

- ❖ Put the tray with meatballs in the oven and bake them for 10 minutes.
- ❖ Meanwhile, make the tomato sauce: in the mixing bowl mix up tapioca flour, crushed tomatoes, and coconut cream.
- ❖ Blend the mixture with the help of the immersion blender until it is smooth and pour in the saucepan.
- ❖ Bring the tomato sauce to boil.
- ❖ After this, pour the sauce over the meatballs and bake the meal for 15 minutes more.

44) SHRIMP SALAD WITH GREENS

Preparation Time: 10 minutes   Cooking Time: 5 minutes   Servings: 4

Ingredients:

- ✓ 1-pound shrimps, peeled
- ✓ 1 tablespoon coconut oil
- ✓ 1 tablespoon lemon juice
- ✓ 1 teaspoon dried cilantro
- ✓ 1 teaspoon dried oregano

Ingredients:

- ✓ ½ teaspoon salt
- ✓ 1 cup lettuce, chopped
- ✓ 1 cup arugula, chopped
- ✓ 1 green pepper, chopped
- ✓ 1 tablespoon olive oil

Directions:

- ❖ In the mixing bowl mix up shrimps and salt.
- ❖ Add dried cilantro and oregano. Mix up the shrimps.
- ❖ Preheat the skillet well and line it with coconut oil.
- ❖ Put the shrimps in the hot skillet and cook for 2 minutes from each side over the medium-low heat.

- ❖ Meanwhile, in the salad bowl mix up lettuce, arugula, and green pepper.
- ❖ Add lemon juice and olive oil. Mix up the salad.
- ❖ Add the cooked hot shrimps.
- ❖ Shake the salad directly before serving.

45) BROCCOLI AND VEAL SALAD

Preparation Time: 10 minutes   Cooking Time: 5 minutes   Servings: 4

Ingredients:

- ✓ 8 oz veal, boneless, chopped, boiled
- ✓ 1 cup broccoli, chopped
- ✓ ½ cup of water
- ✓ 1 teaspoon pine nuts

Ingredients:

- ✓ 1 tablespoon olive oil
- ✓ 1 teaspoon lime juice
- ✓ 1 teaspoon chili powder
- ✓ ½ teaspoon salt

Directions:

- ❖ Pour water in the pan. Add broccoli and bring it to boil. Boil the vegetables for 2 minutes.
- ❖ Then remove them from the hot water and cool in the ice water.
- ❖ Transfer the cooked broccoli in the salad bowl.
- ❖ Add chopped veal, pine nuts, olive oil, lime juice, and chili powder.
- ❖ Then add salt and mix up the salad.

46) LEMON CHICKEN THIGHS

Preparation Time: 15 minutes   Cooking Time: 40   minutes   Servings: 4

Ingredients:

- ✓ 8 chicken thighs, skinless, boneless
- ✓ ½ lemon, sliced
- ✓ 1 teaspoon ground black pepper
- ✓ 1 tablespoon coconut oil
- ✓ 1 teaspoon dried parsley

Ingredients:

- ✓ ½ teaspoon salt
- ✓ 1 teaspoon chili flakes
- ✓ ½ teaspoon garlic powder
- ✓ ¼ cup of coconut milk

Directions:

- ❖ In the mixing bowl mix up garlic powder, chili flakes, salt, dried parsley, and ground black pepper.
- ❖ Then rub the chicken thighs with the spice mixture and leave for 10 minutes to marinate.
- ❖ After this, grease the baking pan with coconut oil.
- ❖ Put the chicken thighs in the prepared baking pan and top with the sliced lemon and coconut milk.
- ❖ Preheat the oven to 365F.
- ❖ Put the baking pan with chicken in the preheated oven and cook for 40 minutes.

47) CHICKEN SALAD WITH CUCUMBERS

Preparation Time: 15 minutes   Cooking Time: 0 minutes   Servings: 2

Ingredients:

- ✓ 10 oz chicken breast, skinless, boneless, boiled
- ✓ 2 cucumbers, chopped
- ✓ 2 tablespoons coconut yogurt

Ingredients:

- ✓ 1 teaspoon fresh dill, chopped
- ✓ 1 teaspoon lemon juice

Directions:

- ❖ Chop the chicken breast on the tiny pieces and put them in the salad bowl.
- ❖ Add chopped cucumbers.
- ❖ After this, in the shallow bowl mix up lemon juice, dill, and coconut yogurt. Whisk the mixture until homogenous.
- ❖ Mix up chicken, cucumbers, and coconut yogurt mixture. The salad is cooked.
- ❖ Store it in the fridge for up to 6 hours.

48) RAINBOW VEGETABLES WITH CHICKEN MEATBALLS

Preparation Time: 20 minutes   Cooking Time: 45 minutes   Servings: 4

Ingredients:

- ✓ 1 sweet red pepper, sliced
- ✓ 1 zucchini, sliced
- ✓ 2 tomatoes, sliced
- ✓ 1 eggplant, sliced
- ✓ 2 cups ground chicken
- ✓ 1 egg, beaten
- ✓ 1 teaspoon ground black pepper

Ingredients:

- ✓ 1 teaspoon chili flakes
- ✓ 1 teaspoon coconut oil
- ✓ 1 teaspoon dried cilantro
- ✓ 1 teaspoon dried thyme
- ✓ 1 teaspoon sunflower oil
- ✓ 1 teaspoon salt

Directions:

- ❖ In the mixing bowl mix up ground chicken, egg, ground black pepper, dried cilantro, thyme, and salt.
- ❖ Then make the small meatballs from the chicken mixture.
- ❖ Grease the baking pan with the coconut oil.
- ❖ Put the zucchini, sweet red pepper, tomatoes, and eggplant in the greased baking pan one-by-one.
- ❖ Put the chicken meatballs in the center of the vegetable mixture.
- ❖ Then sprinkle the meal with sunflower oil and chili flakes.
- ❖ Preheat the oven to 365F.
- ❖ Put the baking pan with the meal in the oven and cook it for 45 minutes.

49) BEEF TOMATO SOUP

Preparation Time: 10 minutes   Cooking Time: 40 minutes   Servings: 4

Ingredients:

- ✓ 2 cups of water
- ✓ 1 cup beef broth
- ✓ ½ cup tomato juice
- ✓ 1 teaspoon tomato paste
- ✓ 1 teaspoon salt

Ingredients:

- ✓ 1 teaspoon ground black pepper
- ✓ ½ cup cauliflower, chopped
- ✓ 1 teaspoon olive oil
- ✓ 8 oz beef shank, chopped
- ✓ ½ teaspoon dried cilantro

Directions:

- ❖ Mix up tomato juice and tomato paste. When the liquid is smooth, pour it in the pan and bring to boil.
- ❖ Add beef shank, beef broth, and water. Close the lid and simmer the mixture over the medium heat for 25 minutes.
- ❖ After this, add salt, ground black pepper, and dried cilantro. Cook the soup for 5 minutes more.
- ❖ Then check if the meat is soft and add cauliflower. Cook the soup for 10 minutes more.
- ❖ Then remove the meal from the heat and let it cool to the room temperature.

50) BEEF BOWL WITH FRIED PLANTAINS

Preparation Time: 10 minutes   Cooking Time: 25 minutes   Servings: 3

Ingredients:

- ✓ 1 plantain, sliced
- ✓ 11 oz ground beef
- ✓ ½ teaspoon dried rosemary
- ✓ ¼ teaspoon dried thyme
- ✓ 1 yellow onion, diced

Ingredients:

- ✓ 1 teaspoon sunflower oil
- ✓ 1 teaspoon salt
- ✓ ½ cup black olives, sliced
- ✓ 2 tablespoons coconut cream

Directions:

- ❖ In the bowl mix up ground beef, dried rosemary, thyme, and salt.
- ❖ Pour sunflower oil in the skillet and heat it up.
- ❖ Add onion and cook it for 5 minutes. Stir it from time to time to avoid burning.
- ❖ Then add ground beef mixture and mix up well.
- ❖ Cook it for 10 minutes on the medium heat. Add coconut cream and cook the mixture for 5 minutes more or until it starts to boil.
- ❖ Then transfer the mixture in the serving bowls.
- ❖ Add sliced black olives.
- ❖ Put the sliced plantain in the hot skillet and fry them for 2 minutes from each side.
- ❖ Add the dried plantains in every serving bowl.

51) MEATBALL SOUP

Preparation Time: 15 minutes   Cooking Time: 25 minutes   Servings: 4

Ingredients:

- ✓ 3 cups chicken broth
- ✓ 1 cup ground chicken
- ✓ ½ cup cauliflower, shredded
- ✓ ¼ cup scallions, chopped

Ingredients:

- ✓ 1 teaspoon sunflower oil
- ✓ ½ teaspoon dried cilantro
- ✓ ½ carrot, grated
- ✓ 1 teaspoon salt
- ❖

Directions:

- ❖ In the mixing bowl mix up ground chicken and dried cilantro.
- ❖ Add cilantro and stir the chicken mixture well.
- ❖ Then make the small meatballs from the chicken mixture.
- ❖ Pour the chicken broth in a saucepan and bring it to boil.
- ❖ Add cauliflower and scallions. Cook the ingredients on the medium heat for 5 minutes.
- ❖ Meanwhile, heat up the sunflower oil in the skillet.
- ❖ Add grated carrot in the oil and cook it for 5 minutes.
- ❖ After this, transfer the cooked grated carrot in the chicken broth.
- ❖ Add salt and bring it to boil.
- ❖ Then add the chicken meatballs and close the lid.
- ❖ Cook the soup for 10 minutes over the medium heat.

52) PIZZA SOUP

Preparation Time: 10 minutes   Cooking Time: 25 minutes   Servings: 4

Ingredients:

- ✓ ½ cup ground chicken
- ✓ 4 oz pepperoni, sliced
- ✓ ¼ cup marinara sauce
- ✓ ½ cup mushrooms, sliced
- ✓ ½ onion, diced
- ✓ 1 tablespoon coconut oil

Ingredients:

- ✓ ½ cup tomatoes, crushed
- ✓ ½ teaspoon garlic powder
- ✓ 3 black olives, sliced
- ✓ 3 cups chicken stock
- ✓ ½ teaspoon salt

Directions:

- ❖ In the saucepan mix up ground chicken, pepperoni, marinara sauce, mushrooms, onion, coconut oil, and tomatoes.
- ❖ Cook the ingredients for 5 minutes. Then stir them well and add garlic powder, salt, and chicken stock.
- ❖ Close the lid and cook the soup for 20 minutes.
- ❖ Ladle the cooked soup in the bowls and top with sliced black olives.

53) CURRY ZOODLES SOUP

Preparation Time: 15 minutes   Cooking Time: 20 minutes   Servings: 4

Ingredients:

- ✓ 1 zucchini, trimmed
- ✓ 1 teaspoon curry paste
- ✓ ½ cup coconut cream
- ✓ 1 eggplant, peeled

Ingredients:

- ✓ 3 cups beef broth
- ✓ 1 teaspoon coconut oil
- ✓ 1 onion, diced
- ✓ 1 teaspoon ground turmeric

Directions:

- ❖ Make the zoodles from the zucchini with the help of the spiralizer.
- ❖ Mix up curry paste and coconut cream.
- ❖ Pour the beef broth in the pan and bring it to boil.
- ❖ Add curry mixture and simmer the liquid for 5 minutes over the low heat.
- ❖ Meanwhile, melt the coconut oil in the skillet.
- ❖ Add onion and cook it for 3 minutes over the medium heat or until it is light brown.
- ❖ Then transfer the onion in the beef broth.
- ❖ Add ground turmeric.
- ❖ Chop the eggplant and add it in the beef broth too.
- ❖ Cook the soup for 5 minutes over the medium heat.
- ❖ Then add zucchini zoodles and boil the soup for 3 minutes.
- ❖ Ladle the cooked soup in the bowls.

54) SHRIMP SOUP

Preparation Time: 10 minutes   Cooking Time: 15   minutes   Servings: 3

Ingredients:

- ✓ 3 oz oyster mushrooms, chopped
- ✓ 1 teaspoon dried lemongrass
- ✓ 8 oz shrimps, peeled
- ✓ 1 red sweet pepper, chopped
- ✓ 1 tablespoon sunflower oil

Ingredients:

- ✓ 1 teaspoon salt
- ✓ teaspoon ground paprika
- ✓ 1 carrot, diced
- ✓ ½ cup of coconut milk
- ✓ 1 cup chicken stock

Directions:

- ❖ In the mixing bowl mix up ground paprika, salt, and dried lemongrass.
- ❖ Then pour the chicken stock in the pan and bring it to boil.
- ❖ Add shrimps and boil them for 2 minutes. Remove the mixture from the heat and let it rest.
- ❖ Meanwhile, pour sunflower oil in the skillet and heat it up.
- ❖ Add grated carrot, oyster mushrooms, and sweet pepper.

- ❖ Cook the vegetables for 5 minutes on the medium heat. Stir them from time to time.
- ❖ Then put the vegetables in the shrimp mixture.
- ❖ Put the mixture on the heat and bring it to boil.
- ❖ Add ground paprika mixture and coconut milk.
- ❖ Close the lid and simmer the soup for 5 minutes.

55) BEEF PHO

Preparation Time: 10 minutes   Cooking Time: 8 minutes   Servings: 4

Ingredients:

- ✓ 3 oz shirataki noodles, cooked
- ✓ 1 tablespoon coconut aminos
- ✓ 1 tablespoon lime juice
- ✓ 2 cups beef broth
- ✓ 1 oz green onion tops, chopped
- ✓ 1 garlic clove, peeled

Ingredients:

- ✓ 1 teaspoon fresh ginger, peeled
- ✓ 10 oz beef steak, boiled, sliced
- ✓ 1 tablespoon fresh cilantro, chopped
- ✓ ¼ cup fresh basil, roughly chopped
- ✓ 1 chili pepper, chopped
- ✓ ½ lime, chopped

Directions:

- ✓ Pour the beef broth in the saucepan.
- ✓ Add coconut aminos, lime juice, garlic clove, fresh ginger, and onion tops.
- ✓ Bring the beef broth to boil and simmer for 5 minutes.

- ✓ After this, strain the beef broth and pour it in the serving bowls.
- ✓ Add sliced beef steak, fresh cilantro, basil, chili pepper, lime, and cooked shirataki noodles. The meal is cooked.

56) ZUPPA TOSCANA

Preparation Time: 15 minutes   Cooking Time: 25 minutes   Servings: 3

Ingredients:

- ✓ 1 bacon slice, chopped
- ✓ 10 oz Italian sausages, chopped hand made
- ✓ ¼ teaspoon chili flakes
- ✓ 1 sweet potato, chopped
- ✓ ¼ yellow onion, diced
- ✓ ¼ teaspoon minced garlic

Ingredients:

- ✓ ¼ cup kale, chopped
- ✓ 2 cups chicken stock
- ✓ ½ cup of coconut milk
- ✓ 1 teaspoon salt
- ✓ 1 teaspoon sunflower oil

Directions:

- ❖ Put the sweet potato, diced onion, minced garlic, and chicken stock in the saucepan.
- ❖ Add coconut milk and salt and close the lid.
- ❖ Simmer the mixture for 10 minutes.
- ❖ Meanwhile, pour the sunflower oil in the skillet.
- ❖ Add Italian sausages and chili flakes. Cook them for 5 minutes and stir from time to time.

- ❖ Then put the cooked sausages in the soup and cook it for 5 minutes more over the medium heat.
- ❖ Meanwhile, fry the bacon until it is golden brown.
- ❖ Add the cooked bacon in the soup mixture.
- ❖ Then add kale and cook the soup for 4 minutes more.

57) GARLIC AND ASPARAGUS SOUP

Preparation Time: 15 minutes   Cooking Time: 17   minutes   Servings: 4

Ingredients:

- ✓ 1-pound asparagus, trimmed
- ✓ 1 garlic clove, peeled
- ✓ 1 tablespoon coconut oil
- ✓ 1 white onion, diced

Ingredients:

- ✓ ½ teaspoon salt
- ✓ 1 teaspoon white pepper
- ✓ ¼ cup coconut cream
- ✓ 2 cups chicken broth

Directions:

- ❖ Chop the asparagus roughly and put it in the pan.
- ❖ Add coconut oil and diced onion.
- ❖ Then add coconut oil and fry the ingredients for 4 minutes.
- ❖ Dice the garlic and add it in the asparagus mixture, stir well and cook for 2 minutes more.

- ❖ Then add coconut cream, white pepper, and chicken broth. Stir the soup mixture and close the lid.
- ❖ Cook the soup for 10 minutes over the medium heat.
- ❖ Then let the cooked soup rest for 10 minutes before serving.

58) FLORENTINE SOUP WITH TOMATOES

Preparation Time: 10 minutes   Cooking Time: 20 minutes   Servings: 2

Ingredients:

- ✓ 3 tomatoes, chopped
- ✓ ¼ cup carrot, chopped
- ✓ ½ cup fresh spinach, chopped
- ✓ ½ garlic clove, peeled, chopped
- ✓ 1 shallot, chopped

Ingredients:

- ✓ 1 tablespoon nut oil
- ✓ 1 teaspoon salt
- ✓ ½ teaspoon cayenne pepper
- ✓ ¼ cup of coconut milk
- ✓ 1 cup of water

Directions:

- ❖ Put tomatoes, carrot, spinach, garlic, shallot, nut oil, salt, and cayenne pepper in the saucepan.
- ❖ Fry the mixture on the medium heat for 4 minutes.
- ❖ Then stir it well and add coconut milk and water.
- ❖ Close the lid and simmer the soup for 15 minutes or until or ingredients are soft.
- ❖ Blend the mixture with the help of the immersion blender until you get the creamy texture.
- ❖ Simmer the soup for 1 minute more and then ladle into the bowls.

59) ACORN SQUASH SOUP WITH GINGER

Preparation Time: 10 minutes   Cooking Time: 25   minutes   Servings: 4

Ingredients:

- ✓ 1-pound acorn squash, peeled, chopped
- ✓ 1 teaspoon ginger paste
- ✓ 1 teaspoon ground turmeric
- ✓ 2 oz pancetta, chopped
- ✓ 1 teaspoon olive oil

Ingredients:

- ✓ 2 tablespoons coconut cream
- ✓ 3 cups chicken stock
- ✓ 1 tablespoon fresh cilantro, chopped
- ✓ 1 teaspoon salt
- ✓ 1 red pepper, chopped

Directions:

- ❖ Pour the chicken stock in the pan and add acorn squash, ginger paste, ground turmeric, coconut cream, fresh cilantro, salt, and red pepper.
- ❖ Close the lid and boil the ingredients for 20 minutes on the medium-low heat.
- ❖ Meanwhile, heat up the olive oil in the skillet.
- ❖ Then add chopped pancetta and roast it for 4-6 minutes or until it is light brown.
- ❖ Check if the acorn squash is cooked with the help of the knife.
- ❖ Then blend the mixture into the cream and simmer it for 3 minutes more.
- ❖ Ladle the cooked soup in the bowls and sprinkle with cooked pancetta.

60) LEEK SOUP

Preparation Time: 10 minutes   Cooking Time: 20 minutes   Servings: 3

Ingredients:

- ✓ 1 white onion, diced
- ✓ 1 oz scallions, chopped
- ✓ 6 oz leek, chopped
- ✓ ½ cup cauliflower, chopped
- ✓ 2 cups of water

Ingredients:

- ✓ 1 cup of coconut milk
- ✓ 1 teaspoon lemon juice
- ✓ ½ teaspoon salt
- ✓ ½ teaspoon dried thyme
- ✓ ½ teaspoon ground black pepper

Directions:

- ❖ Put the white onion and leek in the saucepan.
- ❖ Add cauliflower, water, coconut milk, salt, dried thyme, and ground black pepper.
- ❖ Close the lid and cook the ingredients for 15 minutes on the medium heat.
- ❖ Then blend the mixture with the help of the immersion blender until it is smooth.
- ❖ Add scallions and lemon juice and bring the soup to boil.
- ❖ Then remove it from the heat and cool for 5 minutes. Ladle it in the bowls.

61) FISH CHOWDER

Preparation Time: 15 minutes   Cooking Time: 25 minutes   Servings: 4

Ingredients:

- • 5 oz cod, chopped
- • 4 oz shrimps, peeled
- • 2 oz bacon, chopped
- • 1 teaspoon ground paprika
- • 1 teaspoon salt

Ingredients:

- • 4 oz celery root, chopped
- • 1 teaspoon nut oil
- • ½ teaspoon cumin seeds
- • 2 tablespoons coconut cream
- • 3 cups fish stock

Directions:

- ❖ Preheat the nut oil in the skillet.
- ❖ Add chopped bacon and cook it for 5 minutes. Stir it from time to time.
- ❖ Then pour the fish stock in the saucepan and add coconut cream. Bring the liquid to boil.
- ❖ Add ground paprika, salt, celery root, cumin seeds, and simmer the ingredients for 10 minutes.
- ❖ Then add chopped cod and shrimps.
- ❖ Close the lid and cook the chowder for 10 minutes on the medium-low heat.
- ❖ Then add cooked bacon and remove the chowder from the heat.
- ❖ Let the chowder rest for 10 minutes before serving.

62) CHICKEN POT PIE SOUP

Preparation Time: 15 minutes   Cooking Time: 25 minutes   Servings: 4

Ingredients:

- 1-pound chicken breast, skinless, boneless, chopped
- 2 celery stalks, chopped
- 1 onion, diced
- 2 carrots, diced
- 1 sweet potato, chopped
- ¼ cup green peas
- 2 oz cashew, crushed

Ingredients:

- ½ teaspoon thyme
- 1 teaspoon dried parsley
- 1 teaspoon salt
- 1 teaspoon ground black pepper
- 1 tablespoon olive oil
- 4 cups chicken stock

Directions:

- ❖ Put the chicken in the saucepan.
- ❖ Add olive oil and fry it for 2 minutes from each side.
- ❖ Then add chicken stock, ground black pepper, salt, parsley, and thyme.
- ❖ Close the lid and bring the chicken stock to boil.
- ❖ After this, add onion, carrot, and sweet potato.

- ❖ Boil the ingredients for 15 minutes.
- ❖ Then add celery stalk and green peas.
- ❖ Cook the soup for 5 minutes more.
- ❖ Close the lid and remove the soup from the heat. Let it rest for 10 minutes.
- ❖ Ladle the soup in the bowls and sprinkle with crushed cashews.

63) TOMATO GASPACHO

Cooking Time: 0 minutes   Servings: 2

Ingredients:

- 1 cup tomatoes
- ½ cucumber, chopped
- ½ onion, diced
- ½ bell pepper, chopped
- ½ chili pepper, chopped
- 1 garlic clove, peeled, chopped

Ingredients:

- ½ cup of water
- ½ cup tomato juice
- 1 teaspoon sesame oil
- ½ teaspoon salt
- ½ teaspoon white pepper
- 1 cup hot water, for cooking

Directions:

- ❖ Pour hot water in the saucepan and add tomatoes. Boil them over the medium heat for 30 seconds.
- ❖ Then remove the tomatoes from the water, cool little and peel.
- ❖ Chop the tomatoes roughly and put them in the food processor.
- ❖ Add cucumbers onion, bell pepper, chili pepper, garlic cloves water, tomato, and tomato juice in the food processor.

- ❖ Blend the mixture until smooth.
- ❖ Then pour the mixture in the serving bowls.
- ❖ Add salt, sesame oil, and white pepper. Stir the cooked gazpacho gently.

64) BACON CHOWDER

Preparation Time: 10 minutes   Cooking Time: 30 minutes   Servings: 4

Ingredients:

- 3 cups chicken broth
- 3 oz bacon, chopped
- 3 oz celery stalk, chopped
- ½ yellow onion, chopped
- 1 tablespoon coconut oil
- 1 cup sweet potato, chopped

Ingredients:

- ½ cup coconut cream
- 1 teaspoon salt
- 1 teaspoon ground paprika
- ½ teaspoon cayenne pepper

Directions:

- ❖ Put the coconut oil in the skillet and melt it.
- ❖ Then add yellow onion and cook it until it is light brown.
- ❖ Transfer the cooked onion in the pan and add chicken broth.
- ❖ Then add celery stalk, sweet potato, salt, ground paprika, and cayenne pepper.

- ❖ Close the lid and simmer the mixture until the sweet potato is soft.
- ❖ Meanwhile, put the bacon in the skillet and cook it until golden brown.
- ❖ When the sweet potato is soft, add coconut cream in the chowder and bring it to boil.
- ❖ Then add cooked bacon and cook the chowder for 5 minutes more.

65) CABBAGE SOUP

Preparation Time: 10 minutes   Cooking Time: 25 minutes   Servings: 4

Ingredients:

- 1 cup cabbage, shredded
- 1 carrot, diced
- ¼ cup fresh dill, chopped
- 4 chicken drumsticks

Ingredients:

- 1 teaspoon salt
- 1 teaspoon dried oregano
- 1 tablespoon olive oil
- ½ teaspoon chili powder
- 4 cups of water

Directions:

- ❖ Put the chicken drumsticks in the pan and add water.
- ❖ Cook the chicken on the medium heat for 15 minutes.
- ❖ Meanwhile, pour the olive oil in the skillet and add the diced carrot. Cook it until it is light brown.

- ❖ Then add a carrot in the chicken.
- ❖ Add dill, salt, oregano, and chili pepper.
- ❖ Then add cabbage and cook the soup for 10 minutes over the medium heat.

66) CARROT SOUP

Preparation Time: 10 minutes   Cooking Time: 35 minutes   Servings: 4

Ingredients:

- 3 cups carrot, chopped
- 1 cup leek, chopped
- 1 garlic clove, diced
- 1 teaspoon coconut oil

Ingredients:

- 1 teaspoon salt
- 1 apple, chopped
- 4 cups beef broth

Directions:

- ❖ Heat up the coconut oil in the skillet.
- ❖ Then add garlic and leek.
- ❖ Stir the mixture and simmer it for 304 minutes.
- ❖ Then pour the beef broth in the pan and bring to boil.
- ❖ Add chopped apple and carrot. Cook the ingredients for 20 minutes or until the carrot is soft.

- ❖ Then add garlic and salt.
- ❖ Cook the soup for 5 minutes more.
- ❖ Then blend the mixture until smooth with the help of the immersion blender.
- ❖ Simmer the soup for 5 minutes more.

67) MUSHROOM SOUP

Preparation Time: 10 minutes   Cooking Time: 30 minutes   Servings: 2

Ingredients:

- ½ teaspoon ground nutmeg
- ½ teaspoon salt
- ½ teaspoon dried thyme
- ½ teaspoon ground black pepper
- 2 cup chicken stock

Ingredients:

- 1 cup white mushrooms, chopped
- 1 onion, diced
- 1 teaspoon olive oil
- ½ cup coconut cream

Directions:

- ❖ Heat up olive oil in the skillet and add diced onion. Cook it for 3 minutes on the medium heat. Stir it from time to time.
- ❖ Then add chopped mushrooms and cook the ingredients for 5 minutes more. Stir them frequently to avoid burning.
- ❖ Pour the chicken stock in the pan and bring to boil.

- ❖ After this, add coconut cream and cook the vegetables for 10 minutes more
- ❖ Add white mushroom mixture, salt, thyme, ground black pepper, and close the lid.
- ❖ Simmer the soup for 10 minutes.
- ❖ Then blend it until you get the smooth texture and ladle in the serving bowls.

68) MEDITERRANEAN STUFFED PEPPERS

Preparation Time: 20 minutes   Cooking Time: 50 minutes   Servings: 4

Ingredients:

- 4 bell peppers seeded and halved lengthwise
- 1 cup low-sodium vegetable broth
- 1 cup uncooked couscous
- 1/4 teaspoon kosher salt
- 1/4 teaspoon ground turmeric
- 1 tablespoon olive oil
- 1/2 medium yellow onion, chopped

Ingredients:

- 2 cloves garlic, minced
- 1 cup sun-dried tomatoes, drained and chopped
- 1/4 cup sliced black olives
- 1 teaspoon kosher salt
- 1/2 teaspoon black pepper
- 1/4 cup pine nuts
- 1/4 cup fresh basil chopped

Directions:

- ❖ Program your oven to 400F, then grease a 9 x 13-inch baking pan with olive oil or mom-stick spray.
- ❖ Add the vegetable broth to a heavy-bottom saucepan and bring it to a boil over medium-high heat
- ❖ Remove the vegetable broth from the stove and add the couscous, 1/4 teaspoon of salt, turmeric and stir to combine
- ❖ Cover the saucepan with the lid and let the couscous sit for ten minutes until the couscous has absorbed the broth
- ❖ While the couscous is sitting, place one tablespoon of olive oil in a skillet over medium-high heat
- ❖ Add the onion and sauté for 3-4 minutes until it is softened. Stir in the garlic and oregano and cook for a minute until it is aromatic.

- ❖ Then the sundried tomatoes and olives and cook for 1-2 minutes. Add the couscous, pine nuts, basil, salt, and pepper and stir to combine.
- ❖ Fill the halved bell peppers with the couscous filling and place each pepper into the prepared baking dish
- ❖ Cover the Mediterranean stuffed peppers tightly with aluminum foil and bake for 35-40 minutes
- ❖ Then take the foil off and cook 10-15 minutes until the peppers are tender and golden brown on top
- ❖ Serve and enjoy!

69) CURRIED CHICKEN SALAD

Preparation Time: 10 minutes   Cooking Time: 0 minutes   Servings: 3-4

Ingredients:

- 1/2 cup mashed garlic and avocado, at room temperature
- 1 tsp. apple-cider vinegar
- 1/2 lemon, juiced
- 2 tsp. powdered turmeric
- 1 tsp. powdered ginger

Ingredients:

- 1/4 tsp. sea salt
- 1 lb. shredded pastured chicken breast
- 1/4 cup chopped red onion
- 1/4 cup raisins
- 2 tbsp. chopped parsley

Directions:

- ❖ In a bowl, merge together lemon juice, apple cider vinegar, avocado mash, ginger, turmeric and sea salt until well blended.
- ❖ Add chicken breasts, raisins, and red onion; stir to mix well.

- ❖ Garnish with chopped parsley and serve.

70) RATATOUILLE

Preparation Time: 15 minutes   Cooking Time: 60 minutes   Servings: 6

Ingredients:

- 2 zucchini, sliced into 1/4 inch rounds
- 2 yellow squash, sliced into 1/4 inch rounds
- 2 small eggplants, sliced into 1/4 inch rounds
- 5 Roma tomatoes, sliced into 1/4 inch rounds
- 1 26 oz. jar of tomato basil pasta sauce
- 2 teaspoons fresh thyme
- 2 tablespoons fresh basil

Ingredients:

- 2 teaspoon fresh oregano
- 1 teaspoon of minced garlic
- 1 teaspoon paprika
- 1 teaspoon kosher salt
- 1/4 teaspoon black pepper
- 4 tablespoons of olive oil

Directions:

- ❖ Program the oven to 375 F, then pour the pasta sauce into a baking dish
- ❖ Then layer the zucchini, eggplant, and tomato rounds in the dish in a spiral pattern until the baking dish is completely covered.
- ❖ Add the minced garlic, thyme, basil, oregano, paprika, salt, pepper, and olive oil to a small bowl and whisk to combine
- ❖ Pour the garlic herb mixture over the vegetables and cover the ratatouille with aluminum foil.
- ❖ Bake the ratatouille for 35-40 minutes, remove the foil from the ratatouille
- ❖ Bake for an additional 15-20 minutes until the vegetables are tender and soft.

71) BLACK BEAN QUINOA CORN CHILI

Preparation Time: 15 minutes   Cooking Time: 45 minutes   Servings: 10

Ingredients:

- 1 cup uncooked quinoa, rinsed
- 2 cups water
- 1 tablespoon olive oil
- 1 red onion, chopped
- 4 cloves garlic, minced
- 1 tablespoon chili powder
- 1 tablespoon ground cumin
- 1 teaspoon paprika

Ingredients:

- 1 28 oz. can fire-roasted crushed tomatoes
- 2 19 oz. cans black beans, rinsed and drained
- 2 red bell pepper, chopped
- 1 teaspoon dried oregano
- 1 teaspoon kosher salt
- 1/2 teaspoon black pepper
- 1 cup frozen corn

Directions:

- ❖ Place the quinoa and water into a sauce pot and bring it to a boil over medium-high heat
- ❖ Decrease the flame to medium-low, cover the saucepot with the lid
- ❖ Cook the quinoa for 15-20 minutes until it is tender, then set the cooked quinoa aside.
- ❖ While the quinoa is cooking, place the olive oil into a large, heavy-bottom saucepot over medium-high heat
- ❖ Add the red onion, and sauté for 5 minutes until the onion has softened
- ❖ Stir in the garlic, chili powder, cumin, and paprika, and cook for a minute until it becomes fragrant.
- ❖ Then the tomatoes, black beans, red bell peppers, oregano, salt, and pepper
- ❖ Let the chili base gently simmer over medium-high heat, decrease the flame to medium-low
- ❖ Seal the saucepot with the lid, and simmer for 20 minutes.
- ❖ Add the quinoa and frozen corn and stir to combine
- ❖ Cook the chili for 5 minutes until it is thoroughly heated.
- ❖ Serve and enjoy!

72) SESAME GINGER SALMON WITH VEGETABLES

Preparation Time: 20 minutes   **Cooking Time:** 50 minutes   **Servings:** 4

Ingredients:

For Salmon:
- 2 tablespoons olive oil
- 2 tablespoons coconut aminos
- 2 tablespoons rice wine vinegar
- 2 tablespoons sesame oil
- 1 tablespoon honey
- 2 cloves garlic, minced
- 1 tablespoon grated fresh ginger
- 1 tablespoon sesame seeds
- 2 green onions, thinly sliced
- 4 5.oz salmon filets

Ingredients:

For vegetables:
- 1 large head of broccoli, cut into florets
- 2 large carrots cut into 1/2 inch rounds
- 1 lb. button mushrooms, sliced

Directions:

❖ To prepare the honey ginger marinade, whisk the olive oil, coconut aminos, rice wine vinegar, sesame oil, honey, garlic, ginger, sesame seeds, and green onions in a large bowl.

❖ Place the salmon fillets into the honey ginger marinade and let it sit for at least 1 hour or overnight to allow the salmon to absorb the marinade's flavor.

❖ Program the oven to 400F, then lightly grease a 9×13-inch baking dish with nonstick spray

❖ Add the broccoli, carrots, and mushrooms to the prepared baking dish in an even layer

❖ Then place the honey ginger marinated salmon fillets on top of the vegetables and pour the marinade over the salmon

❖ Bake the salmon for 15-20 minutes. Serve and enjoy!

73) LENTIL STEW

Preparation Time: 10 minutes   **Cooking Time:** 45 minutes   **Servings:** 6

Ingredients:
- 2 tablespoons olive oil
- 1 onion, chopped
- 2 garlic cloves, minced
- 1 large carrot, diced
- 2 cups dried lentils, rinsed
- 1 14 oz, can diced fire-roasted tomatoes
- 6 cup low-sodium vegetable broth

Ingredients:
- 1/2 teaspoon cumin
- 1 1/2 teaspoon smoked paprika
- 2 bay leaves
- 1 teaspoon kosher salt
- 1/2 teaspoon black pepper
- Juice and zest of 1 lemon

Directions:

❖ Place the olive oil into a large saucepot over medium-low heat

❖ Once it is hot, add the onion, cook for 2 minutes. Stir in the carrots and garlic

❖ Then cook for 8-10 minutes until the onions are caramelized.

❖ Add the lentils, tomatoes, vegetable broth, cumin, smoked paprika, bay leaves, salt, and pepper and stir to combine

❖ Turn up the heat to medium-high and bring the lentil stew to a boil.

❖ Cover the saucepot with the lid, decrease the heat to medium-low and cook the soup for 35 - 40 minutes

❖ (Until the lentils have softened and are tender)

❖ Stir in the lemon juice and lemon zest.

❖ Serve and enjoy!

74) ROSEMARY COCONUT ALMOND CRUSTED SALMON

Preparation Time: 10 minutes   Cooking Time: 15 minutes   Servings: 4

Ingredients:

For the crusted salmon:

- 4 salmon fillets
- 1/2 cup roasted almonds, coarsely ground in the food processor
- 1/4 cup sesame seeds
- 1/4 cup shredded unsweetened coconut
- 2 sprigs of fresh rosemary
- 2 tablespoons olive oil
- 1 teaspoon kosher salt
- 1/4 teaspoon black pepper

Ingredients:

For the honey limesauce:

- 3 tablespoons honey
- 1 tablespoon lime juice
- 2 tablespoons coconut aminos
- 1 clove garlic, minced

Directions:

- ❖ To make the sauce, place the honey, lime juice, coconut aminos, and minced garlic into a small bowl, whisk to combine, and set aside.
- ❖ To make the salmon combine the almonds, sesame seeds, and shredded coconut in a bowl, then transfer the almond mixture onto a plate.
- ❖ Brush the tops of the salmon fillets with one tablespoon of olive oil
- ❖ Then press the top of each salmon fillet into the almond coconut breading
- ❖ Season each fillet with salt and pepper.
- ❖ Place the remaining tablespoon of olive oil in a large skillet over medium-high heat

- ❖ Once it is hot, place each salmon fillet, crust side down, into the skillet and sear it for 4-5 minutes
- ❖ Check every so often to ensure the crust does not burn
- ❖ Turn the salmon over, and sear it for an additional 5-7 minutes until salmon reaches your preferred doneness.
- ❖ Place the salmon on a serving dish, and drizzle with the honey lime sauce.
- ❖ Serve and enjoy!

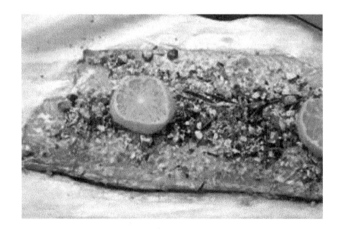

75) SPICY PEANUT CHICKEN STIR- FRY WITH SWEET POTATO NOODLES

Preparation Time: 10 minutes   Cooking Time: 20 minutes   Servings: 4

Ingredients: Ingredients:

For the peanut sauce
- 3 tablespoons all-natural smooth peanut butter
- 2 tablespoons coconut aminos
- 1 teaspoon ginger, minced
- 1 garlic clove, minced
- 1 tablespoon red pepper flakes
- 1/2 tablespoon agave nectar
- 1 teaspoon sesame oil
- 3/4 cup light coconut milk

For the stir fry
- 3 medium sweet potatoes, peeled and spiralized
- 1 pound organic chicken thighs, cut into 1-inch pieces
- 1 teaspoon kosher salt
- 1/2 teaspoon black pepper
- 1 tablespoon sesame oil3 cups broccoli florets
- 2 medium red bell pepper, sliced into thin strips
- 1 large carrot, cut into thin strips

Directions:

- ❖ To make the peanut sauce whisk the peanut butter, coconut aminos, ginger, garlic, red pepper flakes
- ❖ Then agave nectar, sesame oil, and coconut milk in a medium bowl until it is smooth. Set the peanut sauce aside.
- ❖ Generously season the chicken thighs with salt and pepper
- ❖ Place 1/2 tablespoon of sesame oil in a large skillet on medium-high heat
- ❖ When the sesame oil is hot, add the chicken thighs and sauté for 4-6 minutes until the chicken is no longer pink
- ❖ Transfer the chicken thighs to a bowl and set aside.

- ❖ Add 1/2 tablespoon of sesame oil to the skillet, then add the broccoli florets, red pepper strips, and carrots
- ❖ Sauté the vegetables for 5 minutes until the broccoli and carrots are semi-tender. Add the spiralized sweet potato and cook for 2-3 minutes.
- ❖ Pour the peanut sauce and add the chicken to the pot, tossing to coat the vegetables in the sauce
- ❖ Decrease the flame to medium-low and cook for another 2-3 minutes until sweet potato noodles are tender.
- ❖ Serve and enjoy!

76) POMEGRANATE LIME QUINOA SALAD

Preparation Time: 15 minutes   Cooking Time: 15 minutes   Servings: 4

Ingredients: Ingredients:

For the salad:
- 2 cups cooked quinoa, cooled
- 1 cup pomegranate seeds
- ¼ cup chopped pecans
- 2 cups arugula

For the vinaigrette:
- juice of 1 lime
- 2 tablespoon extra virgin olive oil
- 1/4 cup pomegranate juice
- 2 cloves garlic, minced
- 1 teaspoon sea salt
- ¼ teaspoon black pepper

Directions:

- ❖ For the salad, add the quinoa, pomegranate, pecans to a bowl, then place the arugula onto a serving platter.
- ❖ For the vinaigrette, whisk the lime juice, extra virgin olive oil, pomegranate juice, garlic, black pepper, and salt in a bowl.
- ❖ Drizzle the lime pomegranate vinaigrette over the quinoa salad

- ❖ Then stir to combine well and pour the salad onto the bed of arugula.
- ❖ Serve and enjoy!

77) COCONUT-CRUSTED COD

Preparation Time: 25 minutes   **Cooking Time:** 10 minutes   **Servings: 4**

Ingredients:

- 24 ounces cod fillets, sliced into small strips
- 2 tbsp. coconut oil
- 1 cup finely shredded coconut
- 2 cups coconut milk

Ingredients:

- 1 1/2 cups coconut flour
- 1/4 tsp. sea salt
- 1 1/2 tsp. ginger powder

Directions:

- ❖ Rinse and debone the fish fillets.
- ❖ In a bowl, combine ginger powder, coconut flour and sea salt; set aside.
- ❖ Add coconut milk to another bowl and set aside.
- ❖ Add shredded coconut to another bowl and set aside.

- ❖ Dip the fillets into coconut milk, then into the flour mixture, back into the milk, and finally into shredded coconut.
- ❖ Add coconut oil to a skillet set over high heat; when melted and hot
- ❖ Add the fish fillets and cook for about 5 minutes per side or until cooked through.

78) MEXICAN CHICKEN SERVED WITH "RICE"

Preparation Time: 10 minutes   **Cooking Time:** 30 minutes   **Servings: 3**

Ingredients:

- 1 pound boneless and skinless grilled chicken breast, diced into small pieces
- 1 medium avocado
- 4 tbsp. Extra virgin olive oil
- 1 can (4 ounce) diced green chilies
  - 1 head cauliflower, trimmed

Ingredients:

- 1 cup celery, finely diced
- 1 medium onion, diced
- A pinch of chili powder, ground cumin and oregano and to taste
- 1 tsp. sea salt
- Salsa, optional

Directions:

- ❖ Warmth extra virgin olive oil in a skillet set over medium heat. Add onion and sauté for about 10 minutes or until tender.
- ❖ Add celery and sauté for 5 minutes more.
- ❖ Process cauliflower in a food processor until you achieve the texture of rice.

- ❖ Stir cauliflower in the onion mixture and cook, covered, for about 10 minutes or until tender.
- ❖ Add chicken, chilies, chili powder, oregano, cumin, and sea salt.
- ❖ Serve topped with salsa and avocado.

79) ASIAN STIR FRY

Preparation Time: 45 minutes   Cooking Time: 10 minutes   Servings: 4

Ingredients:

- 2 tbsp. coconut oil
- 1 pound boneless, skinless chicken breast
- 1 tbsp. honey
- 2 tbsp. Vinegar
- 2 tbsp. toasted sesame oil
- 2 tbsp. arrowroot powder

Ingredients:

- 1 cup sliced zucchini (about 1 small zucchini)
- 4 ounces stemmed and thinly sliced shiitake mushrooms (about 1 cup)
- 1 1/2 cups sliced strips of baby bock Choy
- 1 cup thinly sliced carrots 4 cups sliced broccoli
- 1 cup finely chopped onion 1/2 tsp. Sea salt
- 11/2 cups water

Directions:

- ❖ Clean and pat dry the chicken; cut into small cubes and place them on a plate.
- ❖ Add coconut oil to a skillet set over medium heat to melt.
- ❖ Add onion and sauté for about 10 minutes or until tender and translucent.
- ❖ Add zucchini, mushrooms, bock Choy, and sea salt; sauté for about 5 minutes.

- ❖ Stir in a cup of water and cook, covered, for about 10 minutes or until veggies are wilted.
- ❖ Dissolve arrowroot powder in a bowl with 1/2 cup of water, stirring until well blended.
- ❖ Stir the arrowroot mixture into the veggies and continue cooking for 3 minutes more or until the sauce is thick and glossy.
- ❖ Stir in honey, sesame oil and vinegar. Serve hot.

80) SPICED CHICKEN WITH GRILLED LIME

Preparation Time: 10 minutes   Cooking Time: 40 minutes   Servings: 4

Ingredients:

- 3 pounds bone-in chicken pieces
- 1 tbsp. garlic powder
- 1 tbsp. smoked paprika
- 2 tbsp. coconut sugar

Ingredients:

- 6 limes, halved
- 1 tsp. allspice
- 1 tbsp. Freshly squeezed ground black pepper
- 1/2 tsp. sea salt

Directions:

- ❖ Place limes and chicken pieces in a bowl.
- ❖ In a small bowl, mix together garlic powder, paprika, coconut sugar

- ❖ Then allspice, pepper and salt; pour over the chicken and mix well.
- ❖ Grill the chicken and limes over medium heat for about 20 minutes per side. Serve.

SNACK RECIPES

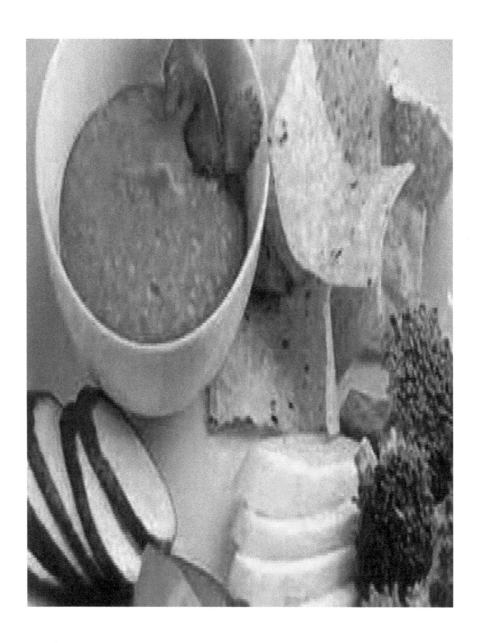

81) CINNAMON AND HEMP SEED COFFEE SHAKE

Preparation Time: 5 minutes   Cooking Time: 0 minutes   Servings: 1

Ingredients:

- ✓ 1 1/2 frozen bananas, sliced into coins
- ✓ 1/8 teaspoon ground cinnamon
- ✓ 2 tablespoons hemp seeds
- ✓ 1 tablespoon maple syrup

Ingredients:

- ✓ 1/4 teaspoon vanilla extract, unsweetened
- ✓ 1 cup regular coffee, cooled
- ✓ 1/4 cup almond milk, unsweetened
- ✓ 1/2 cup of ice cubes

Directions:

- ❖ Pour milk into a blender, add vanilla, cinnamon, and hemp seeds and then pulse until smooth.
- ❖ Add banana, pour in the coffee, and then pulse until smooth.
- ❖ Then ice, blend until well combined, blend in maple syrup and then serve.

82) STRAWBERRY AND BANANA SMOOTHIE

Preparation Time: 5 minutes   Cooking Time: 0 minutes   Servings: 1

Ingredients:

- ✓ 1 cup sliced banana, frozen
- ✓ 2 tablespoons chia seeds
- ✓ 2 cups strawberries, frozen
- ✓ 2 teaspoons honey

Ingredients:

- ❖ 1/4 teaspoon vanilla extract, unsweetened
- ❖ 6 ounces coconut yogurt
- ❖ 1 cup almond milk, unsweetened

Directions:

- ❖ Set all the ingredients in the jar of a food processor or blender and then cover it with the lid.
- ❖ Pulse until smooth and then serve.

83) ORANGE SMOOTHIE

Preparation Time: 5 minutes   Cooking Time: 0 minutes   Servings: 1

Ingredients:

- ✓ 1 cup slices of oranges
- ✓ 1/2 teaspoon grated ginger
- ✓ 1 cup of mango pieces

Ingredients:

- ✓ 1 cup of coconut water
- ✓ 1 cup chopped strawberries
- ✓ 1 cup crushed ice

Directions:

- ❖ Set all the ingredients in the jar of a food processor or blender and then cover it with the lid.
- ❖ Pulse until smooth and then serve.

84) PUMPKIN CHAI SMOOTHIE

Preparation Time: 5 minutes   Cooking Time: 0 minutes   Servings: 1

Ingredients:

- ✓ 1 cup cooked pumpkin
- ✓ 1/4 cup pecans
- ✓ 1 frozen banana
- ✓ 1/4 teaspoon ground cinnamon
- ✓ 1/4 teaspoon cardamom

Ingredients:

- ✓ 1/4 teaspoon ground nutmeg
- ✓ 2 teaspoons maple syrup
- ✓ 1 cup of water, cold
- ✓ 1/2 cup of ice cubes

Directions:

- ❖ Set pecans in a small bowl, cover with water
- ❖ Then let them soak for 10 minutes.

- ❖
- ❖ Drain the pecans, add them into a blender, and then add the remaining ingredients.
- ❖ Pulse for 1 minute until smooth, and then serve.

85) BANANA SHAKE

Cooking Time: 0 minutes

Ingredients:

- ✓ 3 medium frozen bananas
- ✓ 1 tablespoon cocoa powder, unsweetened
- ✓ 1 teaspoon shredded coconut
- ✓ 1 tablespoon maple syrup

Ingredients:

- ✓ 1 tablespoon peanut butter
- ✓ 1 teaspoon vanilla extract, unsweetened
- ✓ 2 cups of coconut water
- ✓ 1 cup of ice cubes

Directions:

- ❖ Add banana in a food processor, add maple syrup and vanilla, pour in water and then add ice.
- ❖ Pulse until smooth and then pour half of the smoothie into a glass.

- ❖ Add butter and cocoa powder into the blender, pulse until smooth, and then add to the smoothie glass.
- ❖ Sprinkle coconut over the smoothie and then serve.

86) GREEN HONEYDEW SMOOTHIE

Preparation Time: 15 minutes   Cooking Time: 15 minutes   Servings: 4

Ingredients:

- ✓ 1 large banana
- ✓ 6 large leaves of basil
- ✓ 1/2 cup frozen pineapple
- ✓ 1 teaspoon lime juice

Ingredients:

- ✓ 1 cup pieces of honeydew melon
- ✓ 1 teaspoon green tea Matcha powde
- ✓ 1/4 cup almond milk, unsweetened

Directions:

- ❖ Set all the ingredients in the jar of a food processor or blender and then cover it with the lid.
- ❖ Pulse until smooth and then serve.

87) SUMMER SALSA

Preparation Time: 5 minutes   Cooking Time: 15 minutes   Servings: 8

Ingredients:

- ✓ 1 cup cherry tomatoes, chopped
- ✓ 1/4 cup chopped cilantro
- ✓ 2 tablespoons chopped red onion
- ✓ 1 teaspoon minced garlic

Ingredients:

- ✓ 1 small jalapeno, deseeded, chopped
- ✓ 1/2 of a lime, juiced
- ✓ 1/8 teaspoon salt
- ✓ 1 tablespoon olive oil

Directions:

- ❖ Set all the ingredients in the jar of a food processor or blender except for cilantro and then cover with its lid.
- ❖ Pulse until smooth and then pulse in cilantro until evenly mixed.
- ❖ Tip the salsa into a bowl and then serve with vegetable sticks.

88) RED SALSA

Preparation Time: 35 minutes   Cooking Time: 15   minutes   Servings: 8

Ingredients:

- ✓ 4 Roma tomatoes, halved
- ✓ 1/4 cup chopped cilantro
- ✓ 1 jalapeno pepper, deseeded, halved
- ✓ 1/2 of a medium white onion, peeled, cut into quarters

Ingredients:

- ✓ 3 cloves of garlic, peeled
- ✓ 1/2 teaspoon salt
- ✓ 1 tablespoon brown sugar
- ✓ 1 teaspoon apple cider vinegar

Directions:

- ❖ Switch on the oven, then set it to 425 degrees F and let it preheat.
- ❖ Meanwhile, take a baking sheet, line it with foil
- ❖ Then spread tomato, jalapeno pepper, onion, and garlic.
- ❖ Bake the vegetables for 15 minutes until vegetables have cooked and begin to brown and then let the vegetables cool for 3 minutes.
- ❖ Transfer the roasted vegetables into a blender, add remaining ingredients and then pulse until smooth.
- ❖ Tip the salsa into a medium bowl and then chill it for 30 minutes before serving with vegetable sticks.

89) PINTO BEAN DIP

Preparation Time: 5 minutes   Cooking Time: 0 minutes   Servings: 4

Ingredients:

- ✓ 15 ounces canned pinto beans
- ✓ 1 jalapeno pepper
- ✓ 2 teaspoons ground cumin

Ingredients:

- ✓ 3 tablespoons nutritional yeast
- ✓ 1/3 cup basil salsa

Directions:

- ❖ Merge all the ingredients in a food processor
- ❖ Cover with the lid and then pulse until smooth.
- ❖ Tip the dip in a bowl and then serve with vegetable slices.

90) SMOKY RED PEPPER HUMMUS

Preparation Time: 5 minutes   Cooking Time: 0 minutes   Servings: 4

Ingredients:

- ✓ 1/4 cup roasted red peppers
- ✓ 1 cup cooked chickpeas
- ✓ 1/8 teaspoon garlic powder
- ✓ 1/2 teaspoon salt
- ✓ 1/8 teaspoon ground black pepper

Ingredients:

- ✓ 1/4 teaspoon ground cumin
- ✓ 1/4 teaspoon red chili powder
- ✓ 1 tablespoon Tahini
- ✓ 2 tablespoons water

Directions:

- ❖ Set all the ingredients in the jar of the food processor and then pulse until smooth
- ❖ Tip the hummus in a bowl and then serve with vegetable slices.

91) SPICY KETCHUP

Preparation Time: 10 minutes   Cooking Time: 15 minutes   Servings: 2

Ingredients:

- ✓ ½ cup tomatoes, chopped
- ✓ ¼ teaspoon chili flakes
- ✓ ¼ teaspoon salt

Ingredients:

- ✓ ¼ teaspoon raw honey
- ✓ 1 teaspoon Italian seasonings
- ✓ 1 tablespoon coconut flour

Directions:

- ❖ Put tomatoes in the saucepan.
- ❖ Add chili flakes, salt, and Italian seasonings.
- ❖ 3Bring the tomatoes to boil and then blend them with the help of the immersion blender until you get the smooth liquid.
- ❖ Add honey and coconut flour and whisk the mixture to get rid of lumps.
- ❖ Simmer the ketchup for 10 minutes on the medium heat.
- ❖ Then pour the cooked ketchup in the glass jar and let it cool.

92) SAUERKRAUT

Preparation Time: 7 days   Cooking Time: 15 minutes   Servings: 4

Ingredients:

- ✓ 1 cup white cabbage, shredded
- ✓ 2 tablespoons salt
- ✓ 1 teaspoon peppercorn

Ingredients:

- ✓ ½ carrot, grated
- ✓ ¼ cup of water

Directions:

- ❖ Put the shredded white cabbage in the big bowl.
- ❖ Add salt and carrot.
- ❖ Mix up the ingredients well and transfer in the big glass jar.
- ❖ Then add peppercorns and water.
- ❖ Close the lid and let the cabbage rest in the warm place for 7 days.

93) BLT BURGER

Preparation Time: 15 minutes   Cooking Time: 15 minutes   Servings: 4

Ingredients:

- ✓ 1 cup ground beef
- ✓ ½ teaspoon ground black pepper
- ✓ ¼ teaspoon chili flakes
- ✓ ½ teaspoon salt

Ingredients:

- ✓ 2 lettuce leaves
- ✓ 1 tomato, sliced
- ✓ 4 bacon slices
  - • 1 teaspoon olive oil

Directions:

- ❖ Put the bacon in the skillet and roast it for 3 minutes from each side or until the bacon is light brown.
- ❖ Then cut every bacon slice on 2 halves.
- ❖ After this, make the burgers: in the mixing bowl mix up ground beef, ground black pepper, chili flakes, and salt.
- ❖ Make 4 burgers from the meat mixture.
- ❖ Pour olive oil in the skillet and add the burgers.
- ❖ Cook them for 5 minutes from each side on the medium heat.
- ❖ Then cut the lettuce leaves into halves.
- ❖ Place the lettuce leaf on the bacon half, then add the burger, and after this, add sliced tomato.
- ❖ Sandwich the ingredients with second bacon half.
- ❖ Repeat the same steps with every burger.

94) PALEO MAYO

Preparation Time: 10 minutes   Cooking Time: 0 minutes   Servings: 10

Ingredients:

- ✓ 1 cup sesame oil
- ✓ 1 egg
- ✓ ¼ teaspoon salt

Ingredients:

- ✓ 1 tablespoon lemon juice
- ✓ 1 teaspoon mustard

Directions:

- ❖ Crack the egg in the mason jar.
- ❖ Add sesame oil, lemon juice, salt, and mustard.
- ❖
- ❖ With the help of the immersion blender blend the mixture until you get the smooth white sauce.

95) SALMON PICKLE BOATS

Preparation Time: 15 minutes   Cooking Time: 0 minutes

Ingredients:

- ✓ 3 pickled cucumbers
- ✓ 1 egg, hard-boiled, peeled
- ✓ 4 oz salmon, canned

Ingredients:

- ✓ 1 teaspoon coconut cream
- ✓ ½ teaspoon minced garlic

Directions:

- ❖ Cut the pickled cucumbers into halves.
- ❖ Then remove the cucumber meat to get the shape of boats.
- ❖ Mix up cucumber meat, canned salmon, coconut cream, and minced garlic in the mixing bowl.
- ❖ Then chop the eggs and add them in the salmon mixture too.
- ❖ Stir the mixture well.
- ❖ Fill the pickled cucumber boats with salmon mixture.

96) SWEET POTATO FRIES

Preparation Time: 10 minutes   Cooking Time: 18 minutes   Servings: 4

Ingredients:

- ✓ 2 sweet potatoes
- ✓ 1 tablespoon sunflower oil

Ingredients:

- ✓ ½ teaspoon dried basil
- ✓ ¼ teaspoon salt

Directions:

- ❖ Peel the sweet potatoes and cut them into the French fries.
- ❖ Then sprinkle the sweet potato fries with dried basil, salt, and sunflower oil.
- ❖ Preheat the oven to 360F.
- ❖ Line the baking tray with baking paper and put the sweet potato fries in it.
- ❖ Flatten them in one layer and transfer in the oven.
- ❖ Bake the sweet potato fries for 18 minutes or until they are light brown.

97) KALE CHIPS WITH ALMOND PARMESAN

Preparation Time: 10 minutes   Cooking Time: 20 minutes   Servings: 6

Ingredients:

✓ 1-pound kale, roughly chopped
✓ 2 oz nut Parmesan, grated

Directions:

❖ Put the chopped kale in the big bowl and sprinkle with salt and sunflower oil.
❖ Then add nut Parmesan and shale the kale well.
❖ After this, preheat the oven to 375F.

Ingredients:

✓ ½ teaspoon salt
✓ ● tablespoon sunflower oil

❖
❖ Line the baking tray with baking paper and put kale inside.
❖ Flatten it well and transfer in the oven.
❖ Bake the chips for 20 minutes. Shake them every 3 minutes to avoid burning.

98) HARD-BOILED EGGS WITH CHILI FLAKES

Preparation Time: 10 minutes   Cooking Time: 7 minutes   Servings: 2

Ingredients:

✓ 2 eggs
✓ 1 teaspoon chili flakes

Directions:

❖ Pour water in the pan and add eggs.
❖ 2.   Boil them for 7 minutes and then cool under cold water.
❖ 3.   After this, peel the eggs and cut into halves.
❖ 4.   Then remove the egg yolks and put them in the bowl.

Ingredients:

✓ 1 teaspoon mustard
✓ 1 cup of water

❖ 5.   Add mustard and chili flakes.
❖ 6.   Churn the mixture until smooth.
❖ 7.   After this, fill the egg whites with mustard egg yolks.

99) CARROT FRIES

Preparation Time: 10 minutes   Cooking Time: 10 minutes   Servings: 4

Ingredients:

✓ 2 carrots, peeled
✓ 1 tablespoon coconut oil

Directions:

❖ Cut the carrots on the French fries and sprinkle with dill.
❖ Then put the coconut oil in the skillet and melt it.

Ingredients:

✓ 1 teaspoon dried dill

❖
❖ Put the carrots fries in the skillet in one layer and roast for 3 minutes from each side on the medium heat.
❖ Then dry the cooked fries with the help of the paper towel.

100) ROASTED NUT MIX

Preparation Time: 10 minutes   Cooking Time: 10 minutes

Ingredients:

✓ 3 pecans, chopped
✓ ½ cup almonds, chopped
✓ ¼ cup walnuts, chopped

Directions:

❖ Heat up the avocado oil in the skillet and add chopped pecans, almonds, walnuts, and hazelnuts.
❖ Add salt and mix up the mixture.

Ingredients:

✓ ½ cup hazelnuts, chopped
✓ 1 tablespoon avocado oil
✓ 1 teaspoon salt

❖ Roast it for 10 minutes on the medium heat. Stir the nut mix frequently.

101) BAKED HOMEMADE BEET CHIPS

Preparation Time: 5 minutes   **Cooking Time:** 15 minutes   **Servings:** 4

Ingredients:

- 4 Medium Beets (Rinsed and Scrubbed)
- 2 teaspoons of Extra-Virgin Olive Oil
- 4 sprigs of Fresh Rosemary

Ingredients:

- 4 sprigs of Fresh Thyme Salt
- Ground pepper

Directions:

- Preheat your oven to 350 degrees.
- Peel your beets and thinly slice them
- Place into a large-sized bowl and toss with your olive oil.
- Set to two rimmed baking sheets in a single layer. Sprinkle with pepper and salt
- Chop up your rosemary and thyme and sprinkle it over your beets.
- Bake until slightly browned. Remove from your oven and allow it to cool
- Chips will become crispier as they cool.
- Serve and Enjoy!

102) BAKED HOMEMADE SWEET POTATO CHIPS

Preparation Time: 5 minutes   **Cooking Time:** 15 minutes   **Servings:** 4

Ingredients:

- 2 Large Sweet Potatoes
- 2 tablespoons of Melted Coconut Oil

Ingredients:

- 2 teaspoons of Dried Rosemary
- 1 teaspoon of Sea Salt

Directions:

- Preheat your oven to 375 degrees.
- Peel your sweet potatoes and slice thinly, using your mandolin or a sharp knife
- In a large-sized bowl, toss your sweet potatoes with coconut oil, rosemary, and salt.
- Place your sweet potato chips in a single layer on your rimmed baking sheet covered with parchment paper
- Bake, then flip your chips over and bake for 10 more minutes
- For the last ten minutes, watch your chips closely
- Serve and Enjoy!

103) BAKED HOMEMADE TORTILLA CHIPS

Preparation Time: 5 minutes   **Cooking Time:** 20 minutes   **Servings:** 2

Ingredients:

- 1 Cup of Almond Flour
- 1 Egg White
- 1/2 teaspoon of Cumin
- 1/2 teaspoon of Chili Powder

Ingredients:

- 1/2 teaspoon of Garlic Powder
- 1/4 teaspoon of Paprika
- 1/4 teaspoon of Onion Powder
- 1/2 teaspoon of Salt

Directions:

- Preheat your oven to 325 degrees. In a large-sized bowl
- Combine all of your ingredients together until they form even dough.
- Roll out your dough between two pieces of parchment paper, as thinly as possible
- Remove your top layer of parchment paper. Cut your dough into desired shapes for chips.
- Move your dough, with the parchment paper, onto your baking sheet
- Bake for approximately 11 to 13 minutes, until golden brown
- Remove from your oven and allow to cool for 5 minutes
- Use your spatula to remove the chips from your paper
- Serve and Enjoy!

104) PALEO KALE CHIPS

Preparation Time: 5 minutes   Cooking Time: 15 minutes   Servings: 2

Ingredients:

- 1 bunch of Kale (Washed and Dried)
- 2 tablespoons of Olive Oil

Ingredients:

- Salt

Directions:

- ❖ Preheat your oven to 300 degrees
- ❖ Remove your center stems and either tear or cut up your leaves.
- ❖ Toss your kale and olive oil together in a large-sized bowl
- ❖ Sprinkle with salt. Spread on your baking sheet (or two, depending on the amount of kale)
- ❖ Bake until crisp. Serve and Enjoy!

105) PALEO PUMPKIN PIE BITES

Preparation Time: 5 minutes   Cooking Time: 15 minutes   Servings: 16

Ingredients:

- 1 cup of Pitted Medjool Dates
- 1/4 cup of Unsweetened Coconut Flakes
- 1/2 cup of Pecans
- 2 teaspoons of Vanilla

Ingredients:

- 1/3 cup of Pumpkin Puree
- 1/4 teaspoon of Nutmeg
- 1 teaspoon of Cinnamon
- 1/4 teaspoon of Ground Cloves
- Pinch of Salt

Directions:

- ❖ Place your dates into a small-sized bowl and cover with water
- ❖ Allow to soak for approximately 10 minutes, then drain.
- ❖ Place your pecans into your food processor and pulse until finely ground
- ❖ Attach in the rest of the ingredients, including your soaked dates
- ❖ Pulse until well combined. Adjust your spices to taste
- ❖ Place into your refrigerator for approximately 30 minutes to chill.
- ❖ With your hands form the dough into small-sized balls
- ❖ Serve and Enjoy!

106) STRAWBERRY HOMEMADE FRUIT LEATHER

Preparation Time: 5 minutes   Cooking Time: 15 minutes   Servings: 12

Ingredients:

- 4 cups of Strawberries (Hulled and Chopped)

Ingredients:

- 2 tablespoons of Honey

Directions:

- ❖ Warmth your oven to 170 degrees or the lowest oven temperature setting
- ❖ Line your baking sheet with parchment paper
- ❖ Place your strawberries in a medium-sized saucepan and cook over a low heat until soft
- ❖ Add in your honey and stir well to combine.
- ❖ Use your immersion blender to puree your strawberries in the saucepan
- ❖ (Or transfer to a blender and puree until smooth)
- ❖ Pour your mixture onto the lined baking sheet
- ❖ Spread evenly with your spatula
- ❖ Bake for approximately 6 to 7 hours, until it peels away from your parchment.
- ❖ Once cooled, peel your fruit leather off the paper and use your scissors to cut your fruit leather into strips.
- ❖ Serve and Enjoy!

107)PALEO PARSNIP FRIES WITH TRUFFLE OIL

Preparation Time: 5 minutes   Cooking Time: 20   minutes   Servings: 3

Ingredients:

- 4 Medium Parsnips (Peeled)
- 2 teaspoons of Truffle Oil
- 2 tablespoons of Extra-Virgin Olive Oil

Ingredients:

- 2 tablespoons of Chopped Parsley
- Salt - Ground pepper

Directions:

- ❖ Preheat your oven to 400 degrees
- ❖ Slice your peeled parsnips into thin fries
- ❖ Toss in your bowl with the olive oil, salt, and pepper
- ❖ Spread out in an even layer on your rimmed baking sheet
- ❖ Bake for approximately 20 minutes.
- ❖ Turn your fries over and place back in the oven

- ❖ Turn up the heat to 450 degrees
- ❖ Bake for an approximately 5 to 10 minutes until crispy
- ❖ Watch closely to make sure that the fries do not burn.
- ❖ Place your fries in a large-sized bowl and toss with your parsley and truffle oil.
- ❖ Serve and Enjoy!

108)PALEO SALSA TOMATO BOWLS

Preparation Time: 5 minutes   Cooking Time: 15   minutes   Servings: 4

Ingredients:

- 4 Medium Ripe Roma Tomatoes
- 1/4 cup of Finely Diced Onion
- 1/4 cup of Sliced Black Olives
- 1/2 Jalapeno (Seeded and Finely Chopped
- 1/2 Green Bell Pepper

Ingredients:

- 1 tablespoon of Chopped Fresh Cilantro
- 2 cloves of Minced Garlic
- 2 teaspoons of Balsamic Vinegar
- 1 tablespoon of Grape seed Oil
- Salt and Pepper

Directions:

- ❖ Cut your tomatoes in half
- ❖ In a small-sized bowl, mix together your remaining ingredients
- ❖ Stir together well. Spoon your salsa mixture into your tomato cups

- ❖ Place in the refrigerator to chill.
- ❖ Serve and Enjoy!

109)PALEO DEVILED EGGS

Preparation Time: 5 minutes   Cooking Time: 15   minutes   Servings: 12

Ingredients:

- 6 Eggs
- 1/4 cup of Paleo Mayonnaise
- 3 tablespoons of Finely Chopped Sun-Dried Tomatoes

Ingredients:

- 3/4 teaspoon of Smoked Paprika
- 1/4 teaspoon of Salt
- 1 tablespoon of Chopped Fresh Cilantro

Directions:

- ❖ Place your eggs in your saucepan and cover with cold water
- ❖ Warmth on your stove and bring to a boil
- ❖ Once boiling, turn off your heat and cover. Let stand for approximately 12 minutes.
- ❖ Drain and transfer your eggs to an ice bath for a minute to cool. Peel

- ❖ Slice your eggs in half and scoop the yolks into a bowl
- ❖ Finely mash your yolks. Stir in your mayonnaise, sun-dried tomatoes, paprika, and salt
- ❖ Mix together well. Pipe into your egg white halves, top with cilantro and refrigerate.
- ❖ Serve and Enjoy!

off the shells.

110)CARROTS WITH SESAME SEEDS AND TAHINI PASTE

Preparation Time: 15 minutes   Cooking Time: 0 minutes   Servings: 4

Ingredients:

- 1 cup baby carrot
- 1 tablespoon tahini paste

Ingredients:

- 1 teaspoon sesame seeds

Directions:

- ❖ Wash the baby carrot carefully and peel it if needed.
- ❖ After this, chop the vegetables roughly and put them in the big bowl.
- ❖ Add sesame seeds and sprinkle the carrot with tahini paste.

111)ROASTED BROCCOLI WITH PARMESAN

Preparation Time: 10 minutes   Cooking Time: 10   minutes   Servings: 4

Ingredients:

- 2 head broccolis, cut into florets
- 2 tablespoons extra-virgin olive oil
- 2 teaspoons garlic, minced

Ingredients:

- Zest of 1 lemon Pinch of salt
- ½ cup Parmesan cheese, grated

Directions:

- ❖ Pre-heat your oven to 400 degrees Fahrenheit.
- ❖ Take a large bowl and add broccoli with 2 tablespoons olive oil
- ❖ Then lemon zest, garlic, lemon juice and salt.
- ❖ Spread mix on the baking sheet in single layer and sprinkle with Parmesan cheese.
- ❖ Bake for 10 minutes until tender.
- ❖ Transfer broccoli to serving the dish.
- ❖ Serve and enjoy!

112)SPINACH AND FETA BREAD

Preparation Time: 10 minutes   Cooking Time: 12   minutes   Servings: 6

Ingredients:

- 6 ounces of sun-dried tomato pesto
- 6 pieces of 6-inch whole wheat pita bread
- 2 chopped up Roma plum tomatoes
- 1 bunch of rinsed and chopped spinach
- 4 sliced fresh mushrooms

Ingredients:

- ½ cup of crumbled feta cheese
- 2 tablespoons of grated Parmesan cheese
- 3 tablespoons of olive oil
- Ground black pepper as needed

Directions:

- ❖ Pre-heat your oven to 350 degrees Fahrenheit.
- ❖ Spread your tomato pesto onto one side of your pita bread
- ❖ Place on your baking sheet (with the pesto side up).
- ❖ Top up the pitas with spinach, tomatoes, feta cheese, mushrooms and Parmesan cheese.
- ❖ Drizzle with some olive oil and season nicely with pepper.
- ❖ Bake in your oven for around 12 minutes until the breads are crispy.
- ❖ Cut up the pita into quarters and serve!

113) QUICK ZUCCHINI BOWL

Preparation Time: 10 minutes   **Cooking Time:** 10 minutes   **Servings:** 4

Ingredients:

- ½ pound of pasta
- 2 tablespoons of olive oil
- 6 crushed garlic cloves
- 1 teaspoon of red chili
- 2 finely sliced spring onions

Ingredients:

- 3 teaspoons of chopped rosemary
- 1 large zucchini cut up in half, lengthways and sliced
- 5 large portabella mushrooms
- 1 can of tomatoes
- 4 tablespoons of Parmesan cheese Fresh ground black pepper

Directions:

- ❖ Cook the pasta.
- ❖ Take a large-sized frying pan and place over medium heat.
- ❖ Add oil and allow the oil to heat up.
- ❖ Add garlic, onion and chili and sauté for a few minutes until golden.
- ❖ Add zucchini, rosemary and mushroom and sauté for a few minutes.

- ❖ Increase the heat to medium-high and add tinned tomatoes to the sauce until thick.
- ❖ Drain your boiled pasta and transfer to a serving platter.
- ❖ 8our the tomato mix on top and mix using tongs.
- ❖ Garnish with Parmesan cheese and freshly ground black pepper. Enjoy!

114) HEALTHY BASIL PLATTER

Preparation Time: 25 minutes   **Cooking Time:** 15 minutes   **Servings:** 4

Ingredients:

- 2 pieces of red pepper seeded and cut up into chunks
- 2 pieces of red onion cut up into wedges
- 2 mild red chilies, diced and seeded
- 3 coarsely chopped garlic cloves
- 1 teaspoon of golden caster sugar

Ingredients:

- 2 tablespoons of olive oil (plus additional for serving)
- 2 pounds of small ripe tomatoes quartered up
- 12 ounces of dried pasta
- Just a handful of basil leaves
- 2 tablespoons of grated Parmesan

Directions:

- ❖ Pre-heat the oven to 392 degrees Fahrenheit.
- ❖ Take a large-sized roasting tin and scatter pepper, red onion, garlic and chilies.
- ❖ Sprinkle sugar on top.
- ❖ Drizzle olive oil then season with pepper and salt.
- ❖ Roast the veggies in your oven for 15 minutes.

- ❖ Take a large-sized pan and cook the pasta in boiling, salted water until Al Dente.
- ❖ Drain them.
- ❖ Remove the veggies from the oven and tip in the pasta into the veggies.
- ❖ Toss well and tear basil leaves on top.
- ❖ Sprinkle Parmesan and enjoy!

115)SPICED VEGETABLE COUSCOUS

Preparation Time: 10 minutes   Cooking Time: 20 minutes   Servings: 2

Ingredients:

- Cauliflower 1 head, cut into 1 inch florets
- Extra-virgin olive oil 6 tbsp. plus extra for serving
- Salt and pepper
- Couscous 1 ½ cups
- Zucchini 1, cut into ½ inch pieces
- Red bell pepper 1, stemmed, seeded, and cut into ½ inch pieces

Ingredients:

- Garlic 4 cloves, minced
- Ras el hanout – 2 tsp.
- Grated lemon zest -1 tsp. plus lemon wedges for serving
- Chicken broth 1 ¾ cups
- Minced fresh marjoram 1 tbsp.

Directions:

- ❖ In a skillet, heat 2 tbsp. oil over medium heat.
- ❖ Add cauliflowers, ¾ tsp. salt, and ½ tsp. pepper. Mix.
- ❖ Cover and cook for 5 minutes
- ❖ (Or until the florets start to brown and the edges are just translucent).
- ❖ Remove the lid and cook, stirring for 10 minutes
- ❖ (Or until the florets turn golden brown)
- ❖ Transfer to a bowl and clean the skillet.
- ❖ Heat 2 tbsp. oil in the skillet.
- ❖ Add the couscous. Cook and stir for 3 to 5 minutes
- ❖ (Or until grains are just beginning to brown)
- ❖ Transfer to a bowl and clean the skillet.

- ❖ Heat the remaining 3 tbsp. oil in the skillet
- ❖ Add bell pepper, zucchini, and ½ tsp. salt
- ❖ Cook for 6 to 8 minutes, or until tender.
- ❖ Stir in lemon zest, ras el hanout, and garlic
- ❖ Cook until fragrant (about 30 seconds).
- ❖ Stir in the broth and bring to a simmer. Stir in the couscous
- ❖ Cover, remove from the heat, and set aside until tender (about 7 minutes).
- ❖ Add marjoram and cauliflower; then gently fluff with a fork to combine.
- ❖ Drizzle with extra oil and season with salt and pepper.
- ❖ Serve with lemon wedges.

116)PASTA E FAGIOLI WITH ORANGE AND FENNEL

Preparation Time: 10 minutes   Cooking Time: 30 minutes   Servings: 5

Ingredients:

- Extra-virgin olive oil 1 tbsp. plus extra for serving
- Pancetta 2 ounces, chopped fine
- Onion 1, chopped fine
- Fennel 1 bulb, stalks discarded, bulb halved, cored, and chopped fine
- Celery 1 rib, minced
- Garlic 2 cloves, minced
- Anchovy fillets 3, rinsed and minced
- Minced fresh oregano 1 tbsp.
- Grated orange zest 2 tsp.

Ingredients:

- Fennel seeds ½ tsp.
- Red pepper flakes ¼ tsp.
- Diced tomatoes 1 (28-ounce) can
- Parmesan cheese 1 rind, plus more for serving
- Cannellini beans 1 (7-ounce) cans, rinsed
- Chicken broth – 2 ½ cups
- Water 2 ½ cups
- Salt and pepper
- Orzo – 1 cup
- Minced fresh parsley ¼ cup

Directions:

- ❖ Heat oil in a Dutch oven over medium heat. Add pancetta.
- ❖ Stir-fry for 3 to 5 minutes or until beginning to brown.
- ❖ Stir in celery, fennel, and onion and stir-fry until softened (about 5 to 7 minutes).
- ❖ Stir in pepper flakes, fennel seeds, orange zest, oregano, anchovies, and garlic
- ❖ Cook for 1 minute. Stir in tomatoes and their juice. Stir in Parmesan rind and beans.
- ❖ Bring to a simmer and cook for 10 minutes.
- ❖ Stir in water, broth, and 1 tsp. salt.

- ❖ Increase heat to high and bring to a boil.
- ❖ Stir in pasta and cook for 10 minutes, or until al dente.
- ❖ Remove from heat and discard parmesan rind.
- ❖ Stir in parsley and season with salt and pepper to taste.
- ❖ Drizzle with olive oil and sprinkle with grated Parmesan. Serve

117) SPAGHETTI AL LIMONE

Preparation Time: 10 minutes   Cooking Time: 15 minutes   Servings: 2

Ingredients:

- Extra-virgin olive oil ½ cup
- Grated lemon zest 2 tsp.
- Lemon juice 1/3 cup
- Garlic 1 clove, minced to pate

Ingredients:

- Salt and pepper
- Parmesan cheese 2 ounces, grated
- Spaghetti 1 pound
- Shredded fresh basil 6 tbsp.

Directions:

- In a bowl, whisk garlic, oil, lemon zest, juice, ½ tsp. salt and ¼ tsp. pepper
- Stir in the Parmesan and mix until creamy.
- Meanwhile, cook the pasta according to package directions

- Drain and reserve ½ cup cooking water.
- Add the oil mixture and basil to the pasta and toss to combine.
- Season with salt and pepper to taste and add the cooking water as needed. Serve.

118) SPICED BAKED RICE WITH FENNEL

Preparation Time: 10 minutes   Cooking Time: 45 minutes   Servings: 2

Ingredients:

- Sweet potatoes 1 ½ pounds, peeled and cut into 1-inch pieces
- Extra-virgin olive oil ¼ cup
- Salt and pepper
- Fennel 1 bulb, chopped fine
- Small onion 1, chopped fine
- Long-grain white rice 1 ½ cups, rinsed

Ingredients:

- Garlic 4 cloves, minced
- Ras el hanout 2 tsp.
- Chicken broth 2 ¾ cups
- Large pitted brine-cured green olives ¾ cup, halved
- Minced fresh cilantro 2 tbsp.
- Lime wedges

Directions:

- Adjust the oven rack to the middle position and heat the oven to 400F
- Toss the potatoes with ½ tsp. salt and 2 tbsp. oil.
- Arrange the potatoes in a single layer in a rimmed baking sheet
- Roast for 25 to 30 minutes, or until tender. Stir the potatoes halfway through roasting.
- Remove the potatoes from the oven and lower the oven temperature to 350F.
- In a Dutch oven, heat the remaining 2 tbsp. oil over medium heat.
- Add onion and fennel; next, cook for 5 to 7 minutes, or until softened.

- Stir in ras el hanout, garlic, and rice. Stir-fry for 3 minutes.
- Stir in the olives and broth and let sit for 10 minutes
- Add the potatoes to the rice and fluff gently with a fork to combine.
- Season with salt and pepper to taste.
- Sprinkle with cilantro and serve with lime wedges. Nutrition

119) MOROCCAN-STYLE COUSCOUS WITH CHICKPEAS

Preparation Time: 5 minutes   Cooking Time: 18 minutes   Servings: 2

Ingredients:

- Extra-virgin olive oil ¼ cup, extra for serving
- Couscous 1 ½ cups
- Peeled and chopped fine carrots 2
- Chopped fine onion – 1
- Salt and pepper
- Garlic 3 cloves, minced
- Ground coriander 1 tsp. Ground ginger 1 tsp.

Ingredients:

- Ground anise seed ¼ tsp.
- Chicken broth 1 ¾ cups
- Chickpeas 1 (15-ounce) can, rinsed
- Frozen peas – 1 ½ cups
- Chopped fresh parsley or cilantro ½ cup
- Lemon wedges

Directions:

- ❖ Heat 2 tbsp. oil in a skillet over medium heat.
- ❖ Add the couscous and cook for 3 to 5 minutes
- ❖ (Or until just beginning to brown)
- ❖ Transfer to a bowl and clean the skillet.
- ❖ Heat remaining 2 tbsp. oil in the skillet
- ❖ Add the onion, carrots, and 1 tsp. salt.
- ❖ Cook for 5 to 7 minutes, or until softened.
- ❖ Stir in anise, ginger, coriander, and garlic
- ❖ Cook until fragrant (about 30 seconds).
- ❖ Stir in the chickpeas and broth and bring to simmer.

- ❖ Stir in the couscous and peas.
- ❖ Cover and remove from the heat
- ❖ Set aside for 7 minutes, or until the couscous is tender.
- ❖ Add the parsley to the couscous and fluff with a fork to combine.
- ❖ Drizzle with extra oil and season with salt and pepper.
- ❖ Serve with lemon wedges.

120) VEGETARIAN PAELLA WITH GREEN BEANS AND CHICKPEAS

Preparation Time: 10 minutes   Cooking Time: 35 minutes   Servings: 2

- Ingredients:
- Pinch of saffron Vegetable broth 3 cups
- Olive oil 1 tbsp.
- Yellow onion 1 large, diced
- Garlic 4 cloves, sliced
- Red bell pepper 1, diced
- Crushed tomatoes ¾ cup, fresh or canned
- Tomato paste – 2 tbsp.
- Hot paprika 1 ½ tsp.

- Ingredients:
- Salt – 1 tsp.
- Freshly ground black pepper ½ tsp.
- Green beans 1 ½ cups, trimmed and halved
- Chickpeas 1 (15-ounce) can, drained and rinsed
- Short-grain white rice – 1 cup
- Lemon 1, cut into wedges

Directions:

- ❖ Mix the saffron threads with 3 tbsp. warm water in a small bowl.
- ❖ In a saucepan, bring the water to a simmer over medium heat
- ❖ Lower the heat to low and let the broth simmer.
- ❖ Heat the oil in a skillet over medium heat
- ❖ Add the onion and stir-fry for 5 minutes.
- ❖ Then the bell pepper and garlic

- ❖ Stir-fry for 7 minutes or until pepper is softened.
- ❖ Stir in the saffron-water mixture, salt, pepper
- ❖ Join also paprika, tomato paste, and tomatoes.
- ❖ Add the rice, chickpeas, and green beans
- ❖ Then the warm broth and bring to a boil.
- ❖ Lower the heat and simmer uncovered for 20 minutes.
- ❖ Serve hot, garnished with lemon wedges.

DINNER RECIPES

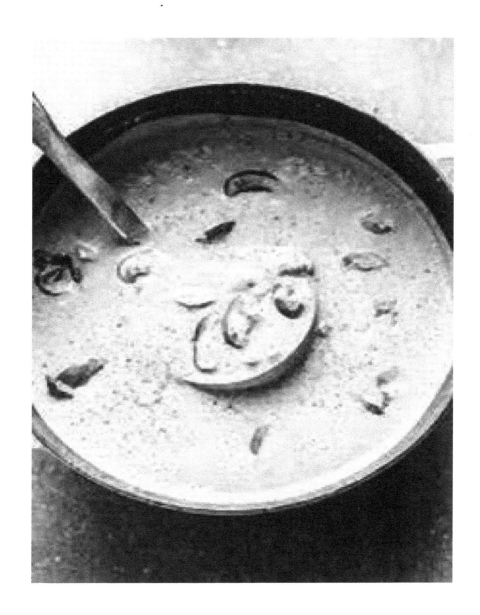

121) RAINBOW CHICKPEA SALAD

Preparation Time: 10 minutes   Cooking Time: 30   minutes   Servings: 4

Ingredients:

- ✓ 16 ounces canned chickpeas, drained
- ✓ 1 medium avocado, sliced
- ✓ 1 bell pepper, seeded and sliced
- ✓ 1 large tomato, sliced
- ✓ 2 cucumber, diced
- ✓ 1 red onion, sliced

Ingredients:

- ✓ 1/2 teaspoon garlic, minced
- ✓ 1/4 cup fresh parsley, chopped
- ✓ 1/4 cup olive oil
- ✓ 2 tablespoons apple cider vinegar
- ✓ 1/2 lime, freshly squeezed
- ✓ Sea salt and ground black pepper, to taste

Directions:

- ❖ Toss all the Ingredients in a salad bowl.
- ❖ Place the salad in your refrigerator for about 1 hour before serving.
- ❖ Bon appétit!

122) MEDITERRANEAN-STYLE LENTIL SALAD

Preparation Time: 10   minutes   Cooking Time: 20   minutes   Servings: 5

Ingredients:

- ✓ 1 ½ cups red lentil, rinsed
- ✓ 1 teaspoon deli mustard
- ✓ 1/2 lemon, freshly squeezed
- ✓ 2 tablespoons tamari sauce 2 scallion stalks, chopped 1/4 cup extra-virgin olive oil 2 garlic cloves, minced
- ✓ 1 cup butterhead lettuce, torn into pieces

Ingredients:

- ✓ 2 tablespoons fresh parsley, chopped
- ✓ 2 tablespoons fresh cilantro, chopped
- ✓ 1 teaspoon fresh basil
- ✓ 1 teaspoon fresh oregano
- ✓ 1 ½ cups cherry tomatoes, halved
- ✓ 3 ounces Kalamata olives, pitted and halved

Directions:

- ❖ In a large-sized saucepan, bring 4 ½ cups of the water and the red lentils to a boil.
- ❖ Immediately turn the heat to a simmer
- ❖ Continue to cook your lentils for about 15 minutes or until tender
- ❖ 4. Drain and let it cool completely.
- ❖ 5. Transfer the lentils to a salad bowl; toss the lentils with the remaining Ingredients until well combined.
- ❖ 6. Serve chilled or at room temperature. Bon appétit!

123) ROASTED ASPARAGUS AND AVOCADO SALAD

Preparation Time: 10 minutes   Cooking Time: 20 minutes   Servings: 4

Ingredients:

- ✓ 1 pound asparagus, trimmed, cut into bite-sized pieces
- ✓ 1 white onion, chopped
- ✓ 2 garlic cloves, minced
- ✓ 1 Roma tomato, sliced
- ✓ 1/4 cup olive oil
- ✓ 1/4 cup balsamic vinegar
- ✓ 1 tablespoon stone-ground mustard

Ingredients:

- ✓ 2 tablespoons fresh parsley, chopped
- ✓ 1 tablespoon fresh cilantro, chopped
- ✓ 1 tablespoon fresh basil, chopped
- ✓ Sea salt and ground black pepper, to taste
- ✓ 1 small avocado, pitted and diced
- ✓ 1/2 cup pine nuts, roughly chopped

Directions:

- ❖ Begin by preheating your oven to 420 degrees F.
- ❖ Toss the asparagus with 1 tablespoon of the olive oil
- ❖ Arrange them on a parchment-lined roasting pan.
- ❖ Bake for about 15 minutes, rotating the pan once or twice to promote even cooking

- ❖ Let it cool completely and place in your salad bowl.
- ❖ Toss the asparagus with the vegetables, olive oil, vinegar, mustard and herbs.
- ❖ Salt and pepper to taste.
- ❖ Toss to combine and top with avocado and pine nuts. Bon appétit!

124) CREAMED GREEN BEAN SALAD WITH PINE NUTS

Preparation Time: 10 minutes   Cooking Time: 10 minutes   Servings: 5

Ingredients:

- ✓ 1 ½ pounds green beans, trimmed
- ✓ 2 medium tomatoes, diced
- ✓ 2 bell peppers, seeded and diced
- ✓ 4 tablespoons shallots, chopped
- ✓ 1/2 cup pine nuts, roughly chopped 1/2 cup vegan mayonnaise

Ingredients:

- ❖ 1 tablespoon deli mustard
- ❖ 2 tablespoons fresh basil, chopped
- ❖ 2 tablespoons fresh parsley, chopped
- ❖ 1/2 teaspoon red pepper flakes, crushed
- ❖ Sea salt and freshly ground black pepper, to taste

Directions:

- ❖ Boil the green beans in a large saucepan of salted water until they are just tender or about 2 minutes.
- ❖ Drain and let the beans cool completely; then, transfer them to a salad bowl.

- ❖ Toss the beans with the remaining ingredients.
- ❖ Taste and adjust the seasonings. Bon appétit!

125) CANNELLINI BEAN SOUP WITH KALE

Preparation Time: 10 minutes   Cooking Time: 25 minutes   Servings: 5

Ingredients:

- ✓ 1 tablespoon olive oil
- ✓ 1/2 teaspoon ginger, minced
- ✓ 1/2 teaspoon cumin seeds
- ✓ 1 red onion, chopped
- ✓ 1 carrot, trimmed and chopped
- ✓ 1 parsnip, trimmed and chopped

Ingredients:

- ✓ 2 garlic cloves, minced
- ✓ 5 cups vegetable broth
- ✓ 12 ounces Cannellini beans, drained
- ✓ 2 cups kale, torn into pieces
- ✓ Sea salt and ground black pepper, to taste

Directions:

- ❖ In a heavy-bottomed pot, heat the olive over medium-high heat
- ❖ Now, sauté the ginger and cumin for 1 minute or so.
- ❖ Now, add in the onion, carrot and parsnip; continue sautéing an additional 3 minutes
- ❖ (Or until the vegetables are just tender)
- ❖ Add in the garlic and continue to sauté for 1 minute or until aromatic.
- ❖ Then, pour in the vegetable broth and bring to a boil

- ❖ Immediately reduce the heat to a simmer and let it cook for 10 minutes.
- ❖ Fold in the Cannellini beans and kale
- ❖ Continue to simmer until the kale wilts and everything is thoroughly heated
- ❖ Season with salt and pepper to taste.
- ❖ Ladle into individual bowls and serve hot. Bon appétit!

126) HEARTY CREAM OF MUSHROOM SOUP

Preparation Time: 10 minutes   Cooking Time: 15 minutes   Servings: 5

Ingredients:

- ✓ 2 tablespoons soy butter
- ✓ 1 large shallot, chopped
- ✓ 20 ounces Cremini mushrooms, sliced
- ✓ 2 cloves garlic, minced
- ✓ 4 tablespoons flaxseed meal

Ingredients:

- ✓ 5 cups vegetable broth
- ✓ 1 1/3 cups full-fat coconut milk
- ✓ 1 bay leaf
- ✓ Sea salt and ground black pepper, to taste

Directions:

- ❖ In a stockpot, melt the vegan butter over medium-high heat.
- ❖ Once hot, cook the shallot for about 3 minutes until tender and fragrant.
- ❖ Add in the mushrooms and garlic and continue cooking until the mushrooms have softened
- ❖ Add in the flaxseed meal and continue to cook for 1 minute or so.

- ❖ 5. Add in the remaining ingredients
- ❖ 6. Let it simmer, covered and continue to cook for 5 to 6 minutes more
- ❖ 7. (Until your soup has thickened slightly)

127) AUTHENTIC ITALIAN PANZANELLA SALAD

Preparation Time: 10 minutes   Cooking Time: 35   minutes   Servings: 3

Ingredients:

- ✓ 3 cups artisan bread, broken into
- ✓ 1-inch cubes
- ✓ 3/4-pound asparagus, trimmed and cut into bite-sized pieces
- ✓ 4 tablespoons extra-virgin olive oil
- ✓ 1 red onion, chopped
- ✓ 2 tablespoons fresh lime juice

Ingredients:

- ✓ 1 teaspoon deli mustard
- ✓ 2 medium heirloom tomatoes, diced
- ✓ 2 cups arugula
- ✓ 2 cups baby spinach
- ✓ 2 Italian peppers, seeded and sliced
- ✓ Sea salt and ground black pepper, to taste

Directions:

- ❖ Arrange the bread cubes on a parchment-lined baking sheet.
- ❖ Bake in the preheated oven at 310 degrees F for about 20 minutes
- ❖ Rotate the baking sheet twice during the baking time; reserve.
- ❖ Turn the oven to 420 degrees F and toss the asparagus with 1 tablespoon of olive oil

- ❖ Roast the asparagus for about 15 minutes or until crisp-tender.
- ❖ Toss the remaining Ingredients in a salad bowl
- ❖ Top with the roasted asparagus and toasted bread.

128) QUINOA AND BLACK BEAN SALAD

Preparation Time: 10 minutes   Cooking Time: 15 minutes   Servings: 4

Ingredients:

- ✓ 2 cups water
- ✓ 1 cup quinoa, rinsed
- ✓ 16 ounces canned black beans, drained
- ✓ 2 Roma tomatoes, sliced
- ✓ 1 red onion, thinly sliced
- ✓ 1 cucumber, seeded and chopped
- ✓ 2 cloves garlic, pressed or minced
- ✓ 2 Italian peppers, seeded and sliced
- ✓ 2 tablespoons fresh parsley, chopped

Ingredients:

- ✓ 2 tablespoons fresh cilantro, chopped
- ✓ 1/4 cup olive oil
- ✓ 1 lemon, freshly squeezed
- ✓ 1tablespoon apple cider vinegar
- ✓ 1/2 teaspoon dried dill weed
- ✓ 1/2 teaspoon dried oregano
- ✓ Sea salt and ground black pepper, to taste

Directions:

- ❖ Place the water and quinoa in a saucepan and bring it to a rolling boil. Immediately turn the heat to a simmer.
- ❖ Let it simmer for about 13 minutes until the quinoa has absorbed all of the water; fluff the quinoa with a fork and let it cool completely. Then, transfer the quinoa to a salad bowl.

- ❖ Add the remaining Ingredients to the salad bowl and toss to combine well. Bon appétit!

129) RICH BULGUR SALAD WITH HERBS

Preparation Time: 10 minutes   Cooking Time: 20   minutes   Servings: 4

Ingredients:

- ✓ 2 cups water
- ✓ 1 cup bulgur
- ✓ 12 ounces canned chickpeas, drained
- ✓ 1 Persian cucumber, thinly sliced
- ✓ 2 bell peppers, seeded and thinly sliced
- ✓ 1 jalapeno pepper, seeded and thinly sliced
- ✓ 2 Roma tomatoes, sliced
- ✓ 1 onion, thinly sliced
- ✓ 2 tablespoons fresh basil, chopped
- ✓ 2 tablespoons fresh parsley, chopped

Ingredients:

- ✓ 2 tablespoons fresh mint, chopped
- ✓ 2 tablespoons fresh chives, chopped
- ✓ 4 tablespoons olive oil
- ✓ 1 tablespoon balsamic vinegar
- ✓ 1 tablespoon lemon juice
- ✓ 1 teaspoon fresh garlic, pressed
- ✓ Sea salt and freshly ground black pepper, to taste
- ✓ 2 tablespoons nutritional yeast
- ✓ 1/2 cup Kalamata olives, sliced

Directions:

- ❖ In a saucepan, bring the water and bulgur to a boil
- ❖ Immediately turn the heat to a simmer and let it cook for about 20 minutes
- ❖ (Or until the bulgur is tender and water is almost absorbed)
- ❖ Fluff with a fork and spread on a large tray to let cool.
- ❖ Place the bulgur in a salad bowl followed by the chickpeas, cucumber, peppers

- ❖ Then tomatoes, onion, basil, parsley, mint and chives.
- ❖ In a small mixing dish, whisk the olive oil, balsamic vinegar
- ❖ Add lemon juice, garlic, salt and black pepper
- ❖ Dress the salad and toss to combine.
- ❖ Sprinkle nutritional yeast over the top, garnish with olives and serve at room temperature

130) CLASSIC ROASTED PEPPER SALAD

Preparation Time: 10 minutes   Cooking Time: 15   minutes   Servings: 3

Ingredients:

- ✓ 6 bell peppers
- ✓ 3 tablespoons extra-virgin olive oil
- ✓ 3 teaspoons red wine vinegar
- ✓ 3 garlic cloves, finely chopped

Ingredients:

- ✓ 2 tablespoons fresh parsley, chopped
- ✓ Sea salt and freshly cracked black pepper, to taste
- ✓ 1/2 teaspoon red pepper flakes
- ✓ 6 tablespoons pine nuts, roughly chopped

Directions:

- ❖ Broil the peppers on a parchment-lined baking sheet for about 10 minutes
- ❖ Rotate the pan halfway through the cooking time, until they are charred on all sides.
- ❖ Then, cover the peppers with a plastic wrap to steam. Discard the skin, seeds and cores.

- ❖ Slice the peppers into strips and toss them with the remaining ingredients
- ❖ Place in your refrigerator until ready to serve

131) POTATO AND CORN CHOWDER

Preparation Time: minutes   Cooking Time: minutes   Servings:

Ingredients:

- ✓ 2 tablespoons low-sodium vegetables broth
- ✓ 1 medium yellow onion, diced
- ✓ 1 stalk celery, diced
- ✓ 1 small red bell pepper, diced
- ✓ 2 teaspoons minced fresh thyme leaves (about 4 sprigs)
- ✓ ½ teaspoon smoked paprika
- ✓ ½ teaspoon no-salt-added Old Bay seasoning
- ✓ 1 jalapeño pepper, deseeded and minced

Ingredients:

- ✓ 1 clove garlic, minced
- ✓ 1 pound (454 g) new potatoes, diced
- ✓ 3 cups fresh corn kernels (about 4 fresh cobs)
- ✓ Salt, to taste (optional)
- ✓ Ground black or white pepper, to taste
- ✓ 4 cup low-sodium vegetable broth
- ✓ 2 teaspoons white wine vinegar Chopped chives, for garnish

Directions:

- ❖ Heat the vegetables broth in a large pot over medium heat. Add the onions and sauté for 4 minutes or until translucent.
- ❖ Add the red bell pepper, celery, paprika, thyme, jalapeño, and Old Bay seasoning
- ❖ Sauté for 1 minutes or until the vegetables are tender.
- ❖ Then the garlic and sauté for another 1 minutes or until fragrant.
- ❖ Join also the corn, potatoes, vegetable broth, salt (if desired), and pepper
- ❖ Stir to mix well. Bring to a boil, then reduce the heat to low

- ❖ Simmer for 25 minutes or until the potatoes are soft.
- ❖ Pour half of the soup in a blender, then process until the soup is creamy and smooth
- ❖ Pour the puréed soup back to the pot and add the white wine vinegar. Stir to mix well.
- ❖ Spread the chopped chives on top and serve.

132) PUMPKIN SOUP

Preparation Time: 20   minutes   Cooking Time: 1 hour 10   minutes   Servings: 8

Ingredients:

- ✓ 3 pounds of quartered seeded sugar pumpkin
- ✓ 3 cups of vegetable broth
- ✓ 2 chopped large shallots
- ✓ 3 chopped fresh sage leaves
- ✓ ¼ cup of Greek yogurt
- ✓ 6 springs of thyme

Ingredients:

- ✓ 1 tablespoon of grated gigger
- ✓ 1/8 teaspoon of nutmeg
- ✓ 1 teaspoon of sea salt
- ✓ Pinch of ground pepper
- ✓ 1 tablespoon of butter
- ✓ 1 ½ tablespoons of olive oil

Directions:

- ❖ Preheat your oven to 450ºF. Spread some oil on a baking sheet.
- ❖ Put pieces of pumpkin on the baking sheet.
- ❖ Drizzle them with olive oil, season with ground pepper and ¼ teaspoon of sea salt. Put thyme sprigs on top.
- ❖ Roast for 1 hour, stirring halfway. Let it cool and remove the skin.
- ❖ Put a large stockpot on medium heat, pour olive oil, and warm it
- ❖ Add chopped shallots and cook for 5 minutes, stirring frequently, until tender.

- ❖ Mix in vegetable broth, pumpkin, sage, and ginger
- ❖ Season with the remaining salt and ground pepper to taste.
- ❖ Bring the mixture to a boil, then remove from the heat.
- ❖ Puree with a blender until smooth consistency
- ❖ Pour in Greek yogurt and blend repeatedly.
- ❖ Serve with some Greek yogurt and enjoy!

133) CANNELLINI PESTO SPAGHETTI

Preparation Time: 5 minutes   Cooking Time: 10 minutes   Servings: 4

Ingredients:

✓ 12 ounces whole-grain spaghetti, cooked, drained, and kept warm

✓ ½ cup cooking liquid reserved

Ingredients:

✓ 1 cup pesto

✓ 2 cups cooked cannellini beans, drained and rinsed

Directions:

❖ Put the cooked spaghetti in a large bowl and add the pesto.

❖ Add the reserved cooking liquid and beans and toss well to serve.

134) CLASSIC TOMATO SOUP

Preparation Time: 10 minutes   Cooking Time: 60 minutes   Servings: 6

Ingredients:

✓ 3 pounds of halved tomatoes

✓ 1 cup of canned crush tomatoes

✓ 2–3 chopped carrots

✓ 2 chopped yellow onions

✓ 5 minced garlic cloves

✓ 2 ounces of basil leaves

✓ 2 teaspoons of thyme leaves

Ingredients:

✓ 1 teaspoon of dry oregano ½ teaspoon of ground cumin

✓ ½ teaspoon of paprika

✓ 2 ½ cups of water

✓ Fresh lime juice, to taste

✓ Extra virgin olive oil Salt, to taste

✓ Black Pepper, to taste

Directions:

❖ Preheat your oven to 450°F. Spread some oil inside a baking sheet.

❖ Mix carrots with tomatoes in a large bowl

❖ Add some oil, salt, black pepper, and toss.

❖ Put the vegetable mixture on the baking sheet in a single layer

❖ Roast for 30 minutes, then set aside for 10 minutes.

❖ Transfer the roasted vegetables in a food processor or a blender, add just a little water, and blend.

❖ Place a large stockpot on medium-high heat, pour 2 tablespoons of olive oil, and warm it.

❖ Add chopped onions and simmer for 3 minutes, then add minced garlic and cook until golden.

❖ Pour the blended mixture into the stockpot.

❖ Add in 2 ½ cups of water, canned tomatoes, thyme, basil, and other seasonings

❖ Bring it to a boil, reduce to low heat, and cover. Simmer for about 20 minutes.

❖ Serve with a splash of lime juice and enjoy!

135) SCALLION AND MINT SOUP

Preparation Time: 5 minutes   Cooking Time: 15 minutes   Servings: 4

Ingredients:

✓ 6 cups vegetable broth

✓ ¼ cup fresh mint leaves, roughly chopped

✓ ¼ cup chopped scallions, white and green parts

Ingredients:

✓ 3 garlic cloves, minced

✓ 3 tablespoons freshly squeezed lime juice

Directions:

❖ In a large stockpot, combine the broth, mint, scallions, garlic, and lime juice

❖ Bring to a boil over medium-high heat.

❖ Cover, reduce the heat to low, simmer for 15 minutes, and serve.

136) KALE AND LENTILS STEW

Preparation Time: 10 minutes   Cooking Time: 50 minutes   Servings: 8

Ingredients:

- ✓ 6 cups (2 pounds) brown or green dry lentils
- ✓ 8 cups vegetable broth or water
- ✓ 4 cups kale, stemmed and chopped into 2-inch pieces
- ✓ 2 large carrots, diced
- ✓ 1 tablespoon smoked paprika

Ingredients:

- ✓ 2 teaspoons onion powder
- ✓ 2 teaspoons garlic powder
- ✓ 1 teaspoon red pepper flakes
- ✓ 1 teaspoon dried oregano
- ✓ 1 teaspoon dried thyme

Directions:

- ❖ In a large stockpot, combine the lentils, broth, kale, carrots, paprika, onion powder
- ❖ Then garlic powder, red pepper flakes, oregano, and thyme
- ❖ Bring to a boil over medium-high heat.

- ❖ Cover, reduce the heat to medium-low, and simmer for 45 minutes
- ❖ Stir every 5 to 10 minutes. Serve warm.

137) LENTIL SOUP WITH SWISS CHARD

Preparation Time: 10 minutes   Cooking Time: 25 minutes   Servings: 5

Ingredients:

- ✓ 2 tablespoons olive oil
- ✓ 1 white onion, chopped
- ✓ 1 teaspoon garlic, minced
- ✓ 2 large carrots, chopped
- ✓ 1 parsnip, chopped
- ✓ 2 stalks celery, chopped
- ✓ 2 bay leaves

Ingredients:

- ✓ 1/2 teaspoon dried thyme
- ✓ 1/4 teaspoon ground cumin
- ✓ 6 cups roasted vegetable broth
- ✓ 1 ¼ cups brown lentils, soaked overnight and rinsed
- ✓ 2 cups Swiss chard, torn into pieces

Directions:

- ❖ In a heavy-bottomed pot, heat the olive oil over a moderate heat
- ❖ Now, sauté the vegetables along with the spices for about 3 minutes until they are just tender.
- ❖ Add in the vegetable broth and lentils, bringing it to a boil.
- ❖ Immediately turn the heat to a simmer and add in the bay leaves

- ❖ Let it cook for about 15 minutes or until lentils are tender.
- ❖ Add in the Swiss chard, cover and let it simmer for 5 minutes more or until the chard wilts.
- ❖ Serve in individual bowls and enjoy!

138) CANNELLINI SOUP WITH KALE

Preparation Time: 5 minutes   Cooking Time: 25 minutes   Servings: 5

Ingredients:

- ✓ 1 tablespoon olive oil
- ✓ 1/2 teaspoon ginger, minced
- ✓ 1/2 teaspoon cumin seeds
- ✓ 1 red onion, chopped
- ✓ 1 carrot, trimmed and chopped
- ✓ 1 parsnip, trimmed and chopped

Ingredients:

- ✓ 2 garlic cloves, minced
- ✓ 6 cups vegetable broth
- ✓ 12 ounces Cannellini beans, drained
- ✓ 2 cups kale, torn into pieces
- ✓ Sea salt and ground black pepper, to taste
- ❖

Directions:

- ❖ In a heavy-bottomed pot, heat the olive over medium-high heat.
- ❖ Now, sauté the ginger and cumin for 1 minute or so.
- ❖ Now, add in the onion, carrot and parsnip; continue sautéing an additional 3 minutes
- ❖ (Or until the vegetables are just tender)
- ❖ Add in the garlic and continue to sauté for 1 minute or until aromatic.

- ❖
- ❖
- ❖ Then, pour in the vegetable broth and bring to a boil
- ❖ Immediately reduce the heat to a simmer and let it cook for 10 minutes.
- ❖ Fold in the Cannellini beans and kale
- ❖ Continue to simmer until the kale wilts and everything is thoroughly heated
- ❖ Season with salt and pepper to taste.
- ❖ Ladle into individual bowls and serve hot

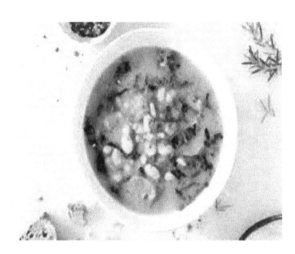

Preparation Time: 10 minutes   Cooking Time: 25   minutes   Servings: 6

Ingredients:

- ✓ 6 ounces dried soba noodles
- ✓ 4 cups vegetable broth, divided
- ✓ 2 cups diced onions
- ✓ 1 cup chopped carrots
- ✓ 1 cup chopped celery
- ✓ 3 garlic cloves, finely diced

Ingredients:

- ✓ ½ teaspoon dried parsley
- ✓ ½ teaspoon dried sage
- ✓ ½ teaspoon dried thyme
- ✓ ½ teaspoon freshly ground black or white pepper (15-ounce) can chickpeas, drained and rinsed
- ✓ ¼ cup chopped fresh parsley, for garnish (optional)

Directions:

- ❖ In a large saucepan, bring 4 cups water to a boil over high heat. Add the soba noodles and cook, stirring occasionally, until just tender, 4 to 5 minutes. Drain in a colander and rinse well under cold water. Set aside.

- ❖ In the same saucepan, heat ¼ cup of broth over medium-high heat. Add the onions, carrots, celery, garlic, parsley, sage, thyme, and pepper and sauté for 5 minutes, or until the carrots are fork-tender.

- ❖ Add the chickpeas and remaining 3¾ cups of broth and bring to a boil. Lower the heat to low, cover, and simmer for 15 minutes.

- ❖ Serve garnished with the parsley, if desired.

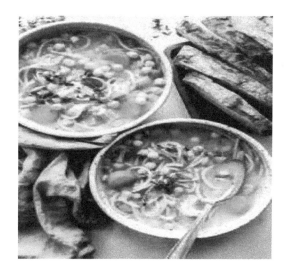

140) VEGAN PHO

Preparation Time: 10 minutes   Cooking Time: 15 minutes   Servings: 6

Ingredients:

- ✓ 1 package of wide rice noodles, cooked
- ✓ 1 medium white onion, peeled, quartered
- ✓ 2 teaspoons minced garlic
- ✓ 1 inch of ginger, sliced into coins
- ✓ 8 cups vegetable broth
- ✓ 1 whole cloves
- ✓ 2 tablespoons soy sauce
- ✓ 1 whole star anise

Ingredients:

- ✓ 1 cinnamon stick
- ✓ 3 cups of water
- ✓ For Toppings:
- ✓ Basil as needed for topping
- ✓ Chopped green onions as needed for topping
- ✓ Ming beans as needed for topping
- ✓ Hot sauce as needed for topping
- ✓ Lime wedges for serving

Directions:

- ❖ Take a large pot, place it over medium-high heat
- ❖ Add all the ingredients for soup in it, except for soy sauce and broth, and bring it to boil.
- ❖ Then switch heat to medium-low level
- ❖ Simmer the soup for 30 minutes and then stir in soy sauce.
- ❖ When done, distribute cooked noodles into bowls
- ❖ Top with soup, then top with toppings and serve.

141) TOMATO TROUT

Preparation Time: 10 minutes   Cooking Time: 50 minutes   Servings: 4

Ingredients:

- 12 oz trout fillet
- 1 cup tomatoes, chopped
- 1 teaspoon ground cumin
- ½ teaspoon ground coriander

Ingredients:

- 1 sweet pepper, chopped
- 1 jalapeno pepper, chopped
- ¼ cup of water
- ½ teaspoon salt

Directions:

- ❖ Cut the trout on 4 servings.
- ❖ In the mixing bowl mix up ground cumin, ground coriander, and salt.
- ❖ Then rub the fish fillets with the spice mixture.
- ❖ Arrange the fish steaks in the saucepan.
- ❖ Add chopped tomatoes, sweet pepper, jalapeno pepper, and water.
- ❖ Close the lid and simmer the fish on the low heat for 50 minutes.

142) MARINATED RAW SALMON

Preparation Time: 10 days   Cooking Time: 10 minutes   Servings: 4

Ingredients:

- 1-pound salmon fillet
- 1 tablespoon salt
- 1 teaspoon ground black pepper
- ½ teaspoon dried thyme
- ½ teaspoon dried rosemary

Ingredients:

- 1 teaspoon cumin seeds
- 1 teaspoon garlic powder
- 1 tablespoon olive oil
- 1 tablespoon lemon juice

Directions:

- ❖ In the mixing bowl mix up salt, ground black pepper, dried thyme, rosemary, cumin seeds, and garlic powder.
- ❖ Then rub the salmon fillet with the spices, sprinkle with olive oil, and lemon juice.
- ❖ Wrap the salmon in the foil and marinate it in the fridge for 10 days.
- ❖

143) SHRIMP JAMBALAYA

Preparation Time: 10 minutes   Cooking Time: 25 minutes   Servings: 2

Ingredients:

- ½ cup cauliflower, shredded
- 1 chili pepper, chopped
- 1 tablespoon olive oil
- ½ teaspoon salt
- 1 teaspoon Cajun seasonings
- 8 oz shrimps, peeled

Ingredients:

- ½ onion, diced
- ¼ zucchini, chopped
- 1 bell pepper, chopped
- 1 tablespoon lime juice
- ½ teaspoon lime zest, grated
- ¼ cup of water

Directions:

- ❖ Pour olive oil in the skillet and heat it up.
- ❖ Add chili pepper and diced onion. Roast the vegetables for 5 minutes on the medium heat.
- ❖ Then add bell pepper and zucchini.
- ❖ Stir the vegetables well and cook for 5 minutes more.
- ❖ After this, add cauliflower, salt, Cajun seasonings, lime juice, and lime zest.
- ❖ Mix up the ingredients.
- ❖ Then add water and shrimps.
- ❖ Close the lid and cook jambalaya for 10 minutes on the medium heat.
- ❖ Stir the meal well before serving.

144)ALMOND BUTTER LOBSTER

Preparation Time: 10 minutes Cooking Time: 10 minutes Servings: 2

Ingredients:

- 4 lobster tails
- 1 tablespoon fresh cilantro, chopped
- ½ teaspoon minced garlic

Ingredients:

- 2 tablespoons almond butter
- 1 bay leaf
- 1 cup water, for cooking

Directions:

- ❖ Pour water in the saucepan and bring it to boil.
- ❖ Add lobster tails and boil them for 5 minutes.
- ❖ After this, remove them from the water and peel.
- ❖ Put the almond butter in the skillet and melt it.

- ❖ Add bay leaf, minced garlic, and fresh cilantro.
- ❖ Cook the ingredients until they start shimmering.
- ❖ Then add peeled lobster tails.
- ❖ Coat the lobster tails in the almond butter mixture well and cook for 1 minute from each side.

145)ORANGE AND SALMON SALAD

Preparation Time: 10 minutes Cooking Time: 5 minutes Servings: 4

Ingredients:

- 10 oz salmon fillet, chopped
- 1 teaspoon coconut oil
- 1 teaspoon ground black pepper
- ½ teaspoon salt
- 2 cups arugula, chopped

Ingredients:

- ½ cup grape tomatoes, halved
- 1 tablespoon lemon juice
- 1 orange, peeled, chopped
- 1 tablespoon olive oil

Directions:

- ❖ Sprinkle the chopped salmon with ground black pepper and salt and put in the skillet.
- ❖ Add coconut oil and roast the salmon for 2 minutes from each side on the medium heat.
- ❖ Then transfer the cooked almond in the salad bowl.

- ❖ Add arugula, grape tomatoes, lemon juice, orange, and olive oil.
- ❖ Shake the salad.

146)RED SNAPPER CURRY

Preparation Time: 10 minutes   Cooking Time: 20 minutes   Servings: 4

Ingredients:

- 12 oz snapper, chopped
- 1 teaspoon curry paste
- 1 cup of water
- 1 chili pepper, chopped
- 1 teaspoon chili flakes

Ingredients:

- 2 shallots, chopped
- 1 tablespoon coconut oil
- 1 teaspoon tomato paste
- ¼ cup coconut cream
- 1 teaspoon fresh cilantro, chopped

Directions:

- ❖ Put the coconut oil in the saucepan and melt it.
- ❖ Add snapper and roast it for 2 minutes from each side.
- ❖ After this, add chili pepper, chopped shallot, and cilantro. Cook the ingredients for 2 minutes.
- ❖ In the separated bowl mix up curry paste, tomato paste, and coconut cream.
- ❖ Add this liquid in the snapper.
- ❖ Then add cilantro, chili flakes, and water.
- ❖ Close the lid and cook the meal for 12 minutes on the medium heat.

147)FENNEL TILAPIA

Preparation Time: 10 minutes   Cooking Time: 15 minutes   Servings: 2

Ingredients:

- 8 oz tilapia fillets (4 oz each tilapia fillet)
- ¼ cup of orange juice
- 1 orange, diced
- 1 tablespoon nut oil

Ingredients:

- ½ teaspoon ground black pepper
- ½ teaspoon tapioca flour
- ¼ teaspoon salt
- ¼ teaspoon fennel seeds

Directions:

- ❖ Pour the nut oil in the skillet and make it hot.
- ❖ Add the fennel seeds in the hot oil and roast them for 1 minute.
- ❖ In the mixing bowl mix up ground black pepper and salt.
- ❖ Then rub the tilapia fillets with ground black pepper mixture and put in the hot nut oil.
- ❖ Roast the fish for 3 minutes from each side.
- ❖ After this, add orange juice and orange.
- ❖ Bring the mixture to boil and add tapioca flour.
- ❖ Stir the meal to avoid flour lumps.
- ❖ Then close the lid and simmer the meal for 10 minutes on the low heat.

148)SMOKED PAPRIKA MACKEREL

Preparation Time: 15 minutes   Cooking Time: 55   minutes   Servings: 8

Ingredients:

- 3-pound mackerel, peeled, trimmed
- 1 tablespoon smoked paprika
- 1 teaspoon ground coriander
- 1 teaspoon onion powder

Ingredients:

- ½ teaspoon salt
- 1 tablespoon olive oil
- ½ teaspoon dried oregano

Directions:

- ❖ In the mixing bowl mix up smoked paprika, ground coriander, onion powder, salt, and dried oregano.
- ❖ Then rub the mackerel with the spice mixture.
- ❖ After this, brush the fish with the olive oil and wrap it in the foil.
- ❖ Preheat the oven to 360F.

- ❖ Put the wrapped mackerel in the oven and cook it for 55 minutes.
- ❖ When the time is over, remove the fish from the oven and discard the foil.
- ❖ Cut the mackerel into the servings.

149)PAN-FRIED SARDINES

Preparation Time: 15 minutes   Cooking Time: 10 minutes   Servings: 4

Ingredients:

- ❖ 1-pound sardines, trimmed
- ❖ ½ cup cassava flour
- ❖ 1 egg, beaten
- ❖ ¼ cup organic almond milk

Ingredients:

- ½ teaspoon salt
- ½ teaspoon chili powder
- 2 tablespoons coconut oil

Directions:

- ❖ Put the sardines in the big bowl and sprinkle with chili powder and salt.
- ❖ In the separated bowl mix up egg and organic almond milk.
- ❖ Dip every sardine in the egg mixture.
- ❖ After this, coat the sardines in the cassava flour.

- ❖ Put coconut oil in the skillet and melt it.
- ❖ Then arrange the sardines in the skillet.
- ❖ Fry the fish for 5 minutes from each side or until it is golden brown

150)SALMON MEATBALLS

Preparation Time: 20 minutes   Cooking Time: 15 minutes   Servings: 2

Ingredients:

- 9 oz salmon fillet
- ½ teaspoon minced garlic
- 1 teaspoon onion powder
- ½ teaspoon dried cilantro

Ingredients:

- 1 teaspoon salt
- 1 egg, beaten
- 1 tablespoon coconut flour
- 1 teaspoon sunflower oil

Directions:

- ❖ Chop the salmon fillet and put it in the blender.
- ❖ Grind the fish until it is smooth and mix up with minced garlic, onion powder, and dried cilantro.

- ❖ Then make the meatballs from the salmon mixture and put them in the baking mold.

Add salt, egg, and coconut flout. Mix up well.

Add the sunflower oil and bake the meatballs for 15 minutes at 360F.

151)CREAMY SPINACH ROTINI SOUP

Preparation Time: 5 minutes   Cooking Time: 15 minutes   Servings: 4

Ingredients:

- 1 teaspoon extra-virgin olive oil
- 1 cup chopped mushrooms
- ¼ teaspoon plus a pinch salt
- 4 garlic cloves, minced, or
- 1 teaspoon garlic powder
- 2 peeled carrots or ½ red bell pepper, chopped
- 6 cups vegetable broth or water

Ingredients:

- Pinch freshly ground black pepper
- 1 cup rotini or gnocchi
- ¾ cup unsweetened nondairy milk
- ¼ cup nutritional yeast
- 2 cups chopped fresh spinach
- ¼ cup pitted black olives or sun-dried tomatoes, chopped
- Herbed Croutons, for topping (optional)

Directions:

- Heat the olive oil in a large soup pot over medium-high heat.
- Add the mushrooms and a pinch of salt. Sauté for about 4 minutes until the mushrooms soften.
- Then the garlic (if using fresh) and carrots, then sauté for 1 minute.
- Add the vegetable broth, then add the remaining ¼ teaspoon of salt

- Join also pepper (plus the garlic powder if using)
- Bring to boil and add the pasta.
- Cook for about 10 minutes until the pasta is cooked. Finish and Serve

152)HOT AND SOUR TOFU SOUP

Preparation Time: 10 minutes   Cooking Time: 15 minutes   Servings: 3

Ingredients:

- 6 to 7 ounces firm or extra-firm tofu
- 1 teaspoon extra-virgin olive oil
- 1 cup sliced mushrooms
- 1 cup finely chopped cabbage
- 1 garlic clove, minced
- ½-inch piece fresh ginger, peeled and minced Salt
- 4 cups water or Vegetable Broth

Ingredients:

- 2 tablespoons rice vinegar or apple cider vinegar
- 2 tablespoons soy sauce
- 1 teaspoon toasted sesame oil
- 1 teaspoon sugar
- Pinch red pepper flakes
- 1 scallion, white and light green parts only, chopped

Directions:

- Press your tofu before you start: Put it between several layers of paper towels
- Place a heavy pan or book (with a waterproof cover or protected with plastic wrap) on top.
- Let it stand for 30 minutes. Discard the paper towels
- Cut the tofu into ½-inch cubes.
- In a large soup pot, heat the olive oil over medium-high heat.
- Add the mushrooms, cabbage, garlic, ginger, and a pinch of salt.

- Sauté for 7 to 8 minutes until the vegetables are softened.
- Add the water, vinegar, soy sauce, sesame oil, sugar, red pepper flakes, and tofu.
- Bring to a boil, then turn the heat to low.
- Finish and Serve
- Simmer the soup for 5 to 10 minutes.
- Serve with the scallion sprinkled on top.

153)WINTER QUINOA SOUP

Preparation Time: 10 minutes   Cooking Time: 25 minutes   Servings: 4

Ingredients:

- 2 tablespoons olive oil
- 1 onion, chopped
- 2 carrots, peeled and chopped
- 1 parsnip, chopped
- 1 celery stalk, chopped
- 1 cup yellow squash, chopped
- 4 garlic cloves, pressed or minced
- 4 cups roasted vegetable broth

Ingredients:

- 2 medium tomatoes, crushed
- 1 cup quinoa
- Sea salt and ground black pepper, to taste
- 1 bay laurel
- 2 cup Swiss chard, tough ribs removed and torn into pieces
- 2 tablespoons Italian parsley, chopped

Directions:

- ❖ In a heavy-bottomed pot, heat the olive over medium-high heat
- ❖ Now, sauté the onion, carrot, parsnip, celery and yellow squash for about 3 minutes
- ❖ (Or until the vegetables are just tender).
- ❖ Add in the garlic and continue to sauté for 1 minute or until aromatic.
- ❖ Then, stir in the vegetable broth, tomatoes, quinoa, salt, pepper and bay laurel
- ❖ Bring to a boil. Immediately reduce the heat to a simmer and let it cook for 1minutes.
- ❖ Fold in the Swiss chard; continue to simmer until the chard wilts.
- ❖ Ladle into individual bowls and serve garnished with the fresh parsley

154)VEGGIE NOODLE SOUP

Preparation Time: 10 minutes   Cooking Time: 15 minutes   Servings: 4

Ingredients:

- 4 celery stalks, chopped into bite-size pieces
- 4 carrots, chopped into bite-size pieces
- 2 sweet potatoes
- 1 sweet onion, chopped into bite-size pieces
- 1 cup broccoli florets
- 1 tomato, diced
- 2 garlic cloves, minced
- 1 bay leaf
- 1 teaspoon dried oregano
- 1 teaspoon dried thyme

Ingredients:

- 1 to 2 teaspoons salt
- Pinch freshly ground black pepper
- 1 cup dried pasta (I prefer a small pasta shape)
- 4 cups DIY Vegetable Stock, or store-bought stock, plus more as needed
- 1 to 11/2 cups water, plus more as needed
- Chopped fresh parsley, for garnishing (optional)
- Lemon zest, for garnishing (optional)
- Crackers, for serving (optional)

Directions:

- ❖ In your Instant Pot, combine the celery, carrots, sweet potatoes, onion, broccol0
- ❖ Then tomato, garlic, bay leaf, oregano, thyme, basil, salt, pepper, pasta, stock, and water
- ❖ Make sure all the good stuff is submerged (add more water or stock, if needed)
- ❖ Close the lid and cooker to High Pressure for 4 minutes (3 minutes at sea level).
- ❖ Once the cook time is complete, release naturally the pressure for 5 minutes; quick release any remaining pressure.
- ❖ Gently remove the lid and stir the soup.
- ❖ Remove and discard the bay leaf and enjoy garnished as desired!

155)CARROT GINGER SOUP

Preparation Time: 10 minutes   Cooking Time: 15   minutes   Servings: 3

Ingredients:

- 7 carrots, chopped
- 1 inch piece fresh ginger, peeled and chopped
- 1/2 sweet onion, chopped
- 1 1/4 cups Vegetable Stock
- 1/2 teaspoon salt

Ingredients:

- 1/2 teaspoon sweet paprika
- Freshly ground black pepper
- Cashew Sour Cream, for garnishing (optional)
- Fresh herbs, for garnishing (optional)

Directions:

- ❖ In your Instant Pot, combine the carrots, ginger, onion, stock, salt, and paprika
- ❖ Season to taste with pepper. Shut down the lid and cook.
- ❖ Once the cook time is processed, let the pressure release naturally for 5 minutes

- ❖ Quick release any remaining pressure.
- ❖ Carefully remove the lid, blend the soup until completely smooth
- ❖ Taste and season with more salt and pepper, as needed. Serve with garnishes of choice.

156)CREAMY TOMATO BASIL SOUP

Preparation Time: 5 minutes   Cooking Time: 15   minutes   Servings: 4

Ingredients:

- 2 tablespoons vegan butter
- 1 small sweet onion, chopped
- 2 garlic cloves, minced
- 1 large carrot, chopped
- 1 celery stalk, chopped

Ingredients:

- 3 cups DIY Vegetable Stock, or store-bought
- 1/4 cup nutritional yeast Salt
- Freshly ground black pepper
- 1 cup nondairy milk

Directions:

- ❖ On your Instant Pot, select Sauté Low
- ❖ When the display reads "Hot," add the butter to melt. Add the onion and garlic
- ❖ Sauté for 3 to 4 minutes, stirring frequently
- ❖ Add the carrot and celery and cook for 1 to 2 minutes more
- ❖ Continue to stir frequently so nothing sticks.
- ❖ Stir in the stock (now is your chance to reincorporate any veggies stuck to the bottom).
- ❖ Add the tomatoes, basil, yeast, and a pinch or two of salt

- ❖ Stir one last time. Shut down the lid and cook.
- ❖ Once the cook time is processed, let the pressure release for 5 to 10 minutes
- ❖ Quick release any remaining pressure.
- ❖ Carefully remove the lid. Blend the soup to your preferred consistency
- ❖ Stir in the milk. Garnish with the remaining fresh basil.

157) CREAM OF MUSHROOM SOUP

Preparation Time: 10 minutes   Cooking Time: 30 minutes   Servings: 4

Ingredients:

- 2 tablespoons vegan butter
- 1 small sweet onion, chopped
- 11/2 pounds white button mushrooms, sliced
- 2 garlic cloves, minced
- 2 teaspoons dried thyme

Ingredients:

- 1 teaspoon sea salt
- 1.3/4 cups DIY Vegetable Stock, or store-bought stock
- 1/2 cup silken tofu
- Chopped fresh thyme, for garnishing (optional)

Directions:

- ❖ On your Instant Pot, select Sauté Low
- ❖ When the display reads "Hot," add the butter to melt.
- ❖ Add the onion. Sauté for 1 to 2 minutes. Then the mushrooms, garlic, dried thyme, and salt.
- ❖ Stir in the stock. Shut down the lid and cook.
- ❖ While the soup cooks, place the tofu in a food processor or blender and process until smooth. Set aside.

- ❖ Once the cook time is processed, let the pressure release naturally for 10 minutes
- ❖ Quick release any remaining pressure.
- ❖ Carefully remove the lid. Using an immersion blender, blend the soup until completely creamy
- ❖ Stir in the tofu, garnish as desired, and it's ready!

158) CURRIED SQUASH SOUP

Preparation Time: 10 minutes   Cooking Time: 41 minutes   Servings: 6

Ingredients:

- 1 tablespoon olive oil
- 1 onion, chopped
- 2 garlic cloves, chopped
- 1 tablespoon curry powder

Ingredients:

- 1 (2- to 3-pound) butternut squash, peeled and cubed
- 4 cups DIY Vegetable Stock, or store-bought stock
- 1 teaspoon salt
- 1 (14-ounce) can lite coconut milk

Directions:

- ❖ On your Instant Pot, select Sauté Low. When the display reads "Hot," add the oil and heat until it shimmers. Add the onion and cook in a low heat.
- ❖ Add the squash, stock, and salt. Shut down the lid and set the cooker to High Pressure for 30 minutes

- ❖
- ❖ Once the cook time is processed, quick release the pressure.
- ❖ Carefully remove the lid. Using an immersion blender, blend the soup until completely smooth. Stir in the coconut milk, saving a little bit for topping when served.

159)MINESTRONE SOUP

Preparation Time: 5 minutes   Cooking Time: 15   minutes   Servings: 7

Ingredients:

- 2 tablespoons olive oil
- 2 celery stalks, sliced 1 sweet onion, diced
- 1 large carrot, sliced, with thicker end cut into half-moons
- 2 garlic cloves, minced
- 1 teaspoon dried oregano
- 1 teaspoon dried basil
- 1/2 to 1 teaspoon salt, plus more as needed

Ingredients:

- 1 bay leaf
- 1 zucchini, roughly diced
- 1 (28-ounce) can diced tomatoes
- 1 (16-ounce) can kidney beans, drained and rinsed
- 1 cup small dried pasta
- 6 cups store-bought stock
- 2 to 3 cups fresh baby spinach
- Freshly ground black pepper

Directions:

- ❖ On your Instant Pot, select Sauté Low. When the display reads "Hot," add the oil, celery, onion, and carrot. Attach the garlic and cook for another minute or so, stirring frequently. Turn off the Instant Pot and add the oregano, basil, salt, and bay leaf. Stir and let sit for 30 seconds to 1 minute.
- ❖ Add the zucchini, tomatoes, kidney beans, pasta, and stock. Shut down the lid and set the cooker to High Pressure for 4 minutes (3 minutes at sea level).
- ❖ Once the cook time is processed, quick release the pressure.
- ❖ Carefully remove the lid, and remove and discard the bay leaf. Stir in the spinach and let it get all nice and wilt. Taste and season with more salt, as needed, and pepper. Serve hot.

160)CARROT-GINGER SOUP

Preparation Time: 5 minutes   Cooking Time: 60   minutes   Servings: 5

Ingredients:

- 2 (10-ounce) packages frozen carrots
- 2 cans diced tomatoes
- 1 medium yellow onion, diced
- 1-piece fresh ginger
- 1.1/2 teaspoons minced garlic (3 cloves)
- Zest and juice of 1 lemon

Ingredients:

- 2 vegetable bouillon cubes
- 3.1/2 cups water
- 2 tablespoons vegan sour cream
- Pinch salt
- Freshly ground black pepper

Directions:

- ❖ Combine the carrots, diced tomatoes, onion, ginger, garlic, lemon zest and juice, bouillon cubes, and water in a slow cooker; mix well
- ❖ Shut down and cook on low heat.
- ❖ Purée using an immersion blender (or with a regular blender, working in batches).
- ❖ Stir in the vegan sour cream and season with salt and pepper.

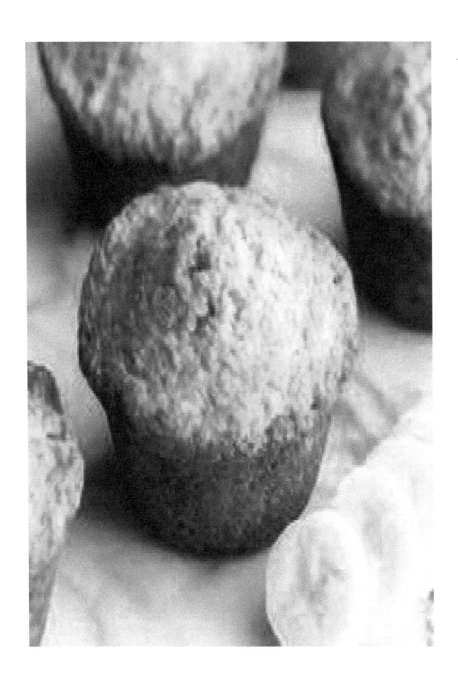

161) RASPBERRY MUFFINS

Preparation Time: 10 minutes   Cooking Time: 25 minutes   Servings: 12

Ingredients:

- ✓   ½ cup and
- ✓   2 tablespoons whole-wheat flour
- ✓   1 ½ cup raspberries, fresh and more for decorating
- ✓   1 cup white whole-wheat flour
- ✓   1/8 teaspoon salt

Ingredients:

- ✓   ¾ cup of coconut sugar
- ✓   2 teaspoons baking powder
- ✓   1 teaspoon apple cider vinegar
- ✓   1 ¼ cups water
- ✓   ½ cup olive oil

Directions:

- ❖   Switch on the oven, then set it to 400 degrees F and let it preheat.
- ❖   Meanwhile, take a large bowl, place both flours in it, add salt and baking powder and then stir until combined.
- ❖   Take a medium bowl, add oil to it, and then whisk in the sugar until dissolved.
- ❖   Whisk in vinegar and water until blended, slowly stir in flour mixture until smooth batter comes together, and then fold in berries.
- ❖   Take a 12-cups muffin pan, grease it with oil, fill evenly with the prepared mixture and then put a raspberry on top of each muffin.
- ❖   Bake the muffins for 25 minutes until the top golden brown, and then serve.

162) CHOCOLATE CHIP CAKE

Preparation Time: 10 minutes   Cooking Time: 50   minutes   Servings: 10

Ingredients:

- ✓   2 cups white whole-wheat flour
- ✓   ¼ teaspoon baking soda
- ✓   1/3 cup coconut sugar
- ✓   2 teaspoons baking powder
- ✓   ½ teaspoon salt
- ✓   ½ cup chocolate chips, vegan

Ingredients:

- ✓   1 teaspoon vanilla extract, unsweetened
- ✓   1 tablespoon applesauce
- ✓   1 teaspoon apple cider vinegar
- ✓   ¼ cup melted coconut oil
- ✓   ½ teaspoon almond extract, unsweetened
- ✓   Cup almond milk, unsweetened
- ❖

Directions:

- ❖   Switch on the oven, then set it to 360 degrees F and let it preheat.
- ❖   Meanwhile, take a 9-by-5 inches loaf pan, grease it with oil, and then set aside until required.
- ❖   Take a large bowl, add sugar to it, pour in oil, vanilla and almond extract, vinegar, apple sauce, and milk, and then whisk until well combined.
- ❖   Take a large bowl, place flour in it, add salt, baking powder, and soda, and then stir until mixed.
- ❖   Stir the flour mixture into the milk mixture until smooth batter comes together, and then fold in 1/3 cup of chocolate chips.
- ❖   Spoon the batter into the loaf pan, scatter remaining chocolate chips on top and then bake for 50 minutes.
- ❖   When done, let the bread cool for 10 minutes and then cut it into slices.
- ❖   Serve straight away.

163) COFFEE CAKE

Preparation Time: 10 minutes   Cooking Time: 45 minutes   Servings: 9

Ingredients:

For the Cake:
- ✔ 1/3 cup coconut sugar
- ✔ 1 teaspoon vanilla extract, unsweetened
- ✔ ¼ cup olive oil
- ✔ 1/8 teaspoon almond extract, unsweetened
- ✔ 1 ¾ cup white whole-wheat flour
- ✔ 2 teaspoons baking powder
- ✔ ½ teaspoon salt
- ✔ ¼ teaspoon baking soda
- ✔ 1 teaspoon apple cider vinegar
- ✔ 1 tablespoon applesauce
- ✔ 1cup almond milk, unsweetened

Ingredients:

For the Streusel:
- ✔ ½ cup white whole-wheat flour
- ✔ 2 teaspoons cinnamon
- ✔ 1/3 cup coconut sugar
- ✔ ½ teaspoon salt
- ✔ 2 tablespoons olive oil
- ✔ 1 tablespoon coconut butter

Directions:

- ❖ Switch on the oven, then set it to 350 degrees F and let it preheat.
- ❖ Meanwhile, take a large bowl, pour in milk, add applesauce, vinegar, sugar, oil, vanilla, and almond extract and then whisk until blended.
- ❖ Take a medium bowl, place flour in it, add salt, baking powder, and soda and then stir until mixed.
- ❖ Stir the flour mixture into the milk mixture until smooth batter comes together, and then spoon the mixture into a loaf pan lined with parchment paper.
- ❖ Prepare streusel and for this, take a medium bowl, place flour in it, and then add sugar, salt, and cinnamon

- ❖ Stir until mixed, and then mix butter and oil with fingers until the crumble mixture comes together.
- ❖ Spread the prepared streusel on top of the batter of the cake and then bake for 45 minutes until the top turn golden brown and cake have thoroughly cooked.
- ❖ When done, let the cake rest in its pan for 10 minutes, remove it to cool completely and then cut it into slices.
- ❖ Serve straight away.

164) CHOCOLATE MARBLE CAKE

Preparation Time: 15 minutes   Cooking Time: 50 minutes   Servings: 8

Ingredients:
- ✔ 1 ½ cup white whole-wheat flour
- ✔ 1 tablespoon flaxseed meal
- ✔ 2 ½ tablespoons cocoa powder
- ✔ ¼ teaspoon salt
- ✔ 4 tablespoons chopped walnuts
- ✔ 1 teaspoon baking powder

Ingredients:
- ✔ 2/3 cup coconut sugar
- ✔ ¼ teaspoon baking soda
- ✔ 1 teaspoon vanilla extract, unsweetened
- ✔ 3 tablespoons peanut butter
- ✔ ¼ cup olive oil
- ✔ 1 cup almond milk, unsweetened

Directions:

- ❖ Switch on the oven, then set it to 350 degrees F and let it preheat.
- ❖ Meanwhile, take a medium bowl, place flour in it, add salt, baking powder, and soda in it and then stir until mixed.
- ❖ Take a large bowl, pour in milk, add sugar, flaxseed, oil, and vanilla, whisk until sugar has dissolved, and then whisk in flour mixture until smooth batter comes together.
- ❖ Spoon half of the prepared batter in a medium bowl, add cocoa powder and then stir until combined.
- ❖ Add peanut butter into the other bowl and then stir until combined.

- ❖ Take a loaf pan, line it with a parchment sheet, spoon half of the chocolate batter in it, and then spread it evenly.
- ❖ Layer the chocolate batter with half of the peanut butter batter, cover with the remaining chocolate batter and then layer with the remaining peanut butter batter.
- ❖ Make swirls into the batter with a toothpick, smooth the top with a spatula, sprinkle walnuts on top, and then bake for 50 minutes until done.
- ❖ When done, let the cake rest in its pan for 10 minutes, then remove it to cool completely and cut it into slices.
- ❖ Serve straight away.

165) CHOCOLATE CHIP COOKIES

Preparation Time: 10 minutes   Cooking Time: 10 minutes   Servings: 11

Ingredients:

- ✓ ¼ cups white whole-wheat flour
- ✓ 1 ½ tablespoon flax seeds
- ✓ ½ teaspoon baking soda
- ✓ ½ cup of coconut sugar
- ✓ ¼ teaspoon of sea salt
- ✓ ¼ cup powdered coconut sugar

Ingredients:

- ✓ 1 teaspoon baking powder
- ✓ 2 teaspoons vanilla extract, unsweetened
- ✓ 4 ½ tablespoons water
- ✓ ½ cup of coconut oil
- ✓ 1 cup chocolate chips, vegan

Directions:

- ❖ Take a large bowl, place flax seeds in it, stir in water and then let the mixture rest for 5 minutes until creamy.
- ❖ Then add remaining ingredients into the flax seed's mixture except for flour and chocolate chips and then beat until light batter comes together.
- ❖ Beat in flour, ¼ cup at a time, until smooth batter comes together, and then fold in chocolate chips.
- ❖ Use an ice cream scoop to scoop the batter onto a baking sheet lined with parchment sheet with some distance between cookies
- ❖ Then bake for 10 minutes until cookies turn golden brown.
- ❖ When done, let the cookies cool on the baking sheet for 3 minutes and then cool completely on the wire rack for 5 minutes.
- ❖ Serve straight away.

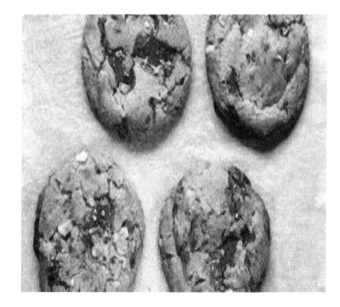

166) LEMON CAKE

Preparation Time: 10 minutes   Cooking Time: 50 minutes   Servings: 9

Ingredients:

- ✓ 1 ½ cup white whole-wheat flour
- ✓ 1 ½ teaspoon baking powder
- ✓ 2 tablespoons almond flour
- ✓ 1 lemon, zested
- ✓ ¼ teaspoon baking soda
- ✓ 1/8 teaspoon turmeric powder
- ✓ 1/3 teaspoon salt
- ✓ ¼ teaspoon vanilla extract, unsweetened
- ✓ 1/3 cup lemon juice

Ingredients:

- ✓ ½ cup maple syrup
- ✓ ¼ cup olive oil
- ✓ ¼ cup of water For the Frosting:
- ✓ 1 tablespoon lemon juice
- ✓ 1/8 teaspoon salt
- ✓ ¼ cup maple syrup
- ✓ 2 tablespoons powdered sugar
- ✓ 6 ounces vegan cream cheese, softened

Directions:

- ❖ Switch on the oven, then set it to 350 degrees F and let it preheat.
- ❖ Take a large bowl, pour in water, lemon juice, and oil, add vanilla extract and maple syrup, and whisk until blended.
- ❖ Whisk in flour, ¼ cup at a time, until smooth, and then whisk in almond flour, salt, turmeric, lemon zest, baking soda, and powder until well combined.

- ❖ Take a loaf pan, grease it with oil, spoon prepared batter in it, and then bake for 50 minutes.
- ❖ Meanwhile, prepare the frosting and for this, take a small bowl, place all of its ingredients in it, whisk until smooth, and then let it chill until required.
- ❖ When the cake has cooked, let it cool for 10 minutes in its pan and then let it cool completely on the wire rack.
- ❖ Spread the prepared frosting on top of the cake, slice the cake, and then serve.

167) BANANA MUFFINS

Preparation Time: 10 minutes   Cooking Time: 30 minutes   Servings: 12

Ingredients:

- ✓ 1 ½ cups mashed banana
- ✓ 1 ½ cups and 2 tablespoons white whole-wheat flour, divided
- ✓ ¼ cup of coconut sugar
- ✓ ¾ cup rolled oats, divided
- ✓ 1 teaspoon ginger powder
- ✓ 1 tablespoon ground cinnamon, divided
- ✓ 2 teaspoons baking powder

Ingredients:

- ✓ ½ teaspoon salt
- ✓ 1 teaspoon baking soda
- ✓ 1 tablespoon vanilla extract, unsweetened
- ✓ ½ cup maple syrup
- ✓ 1 tablespoon rum
- ✓ ½ cup of coconut oil

Directions:

- ❖ Switch on the oven, then set it to 350 degrees F and let it preheat.
- ❖ Meanwhile, take a medium bowl, place 1 ½ cup flour in it, add ½ cup oars, ginger, baking powder and soda, salt, and 2 teaspoons cinnamon and then stir until mixed.
- ❖ Place ¼ cup of coconut oil in a heatproof bowl, melt it in the microwave oven and then whisk in maple syrup until combined.
- ❖ Add mashed banana along with rum and vanilla, stir until combined, and then whisk this mixture into the flour mixture until smooth batter comes together.

- ❖ Take a separate medium bowl, place remaining oats and flour in it, add cinnamon, coconut sugar, and coconut oil and then stir with a fork until crumbly mixture comes together.
- ❖ Take a 12-cups muffin pan, fill evenly with prepared batter, top with oats mixture, and then bake for 30 minutes until firm and the top turn golden brown.
- ❖ When done, let the muffins cool for 5 minutes in its pan and then cool the muffins completely before serving.

168) NO-BAKE COOKIES

Preparation Time: 30 minutes   Cooking Time: 0 minutes   Servings: 9

Ingredients:

- ✓ 1 cup rolled oats
- ✓ ¼ cup of cocoa powder
- ✓ 1/8 teaspoon salt
- ✓ 1 teaspoon vanilla extract, unsweetened

Ingredients:

- ✓ ¼ cup and 2 tablespoons peanut butter, divided
- ✓ 6 tablespoons coconut oil, divided
- ✓ ¼ cup and 1 tablespoon maple syrup, divided

Directions:

- ❖ Take a small saucepan, place it over low heat, add 5 tablespoons of coconut oil and then let it melt.
- ❖ Whisk in 2 tablespoons peanut butter, salt, 1 teaspoon vanilla extract, and ¼ cup each of cocoa powder and maple syrup, and then whisk until well combined.
- ❖ Remove pan from heat, stir in oats and then spoon the mixture evenly into 9 cups of a muffin pan.

- ❖ Wipe clean the pan, return it over low heat, add remaining coconut oil, maple syrup, and peanut butter, stir until combined, and then cook for 2 minutes until thoroughly warmed.
- ❖ Drizzle the peanut butter sauce over the oat mixture in the muffin pan and then let it freeze for 20 minutes or more until set.
- ❖ Serve straight away.

169) PEANUT BUTTER AND OAT BARS

Preparation Time: 40 minutes   Cooking Time: 8 minutes   Servings: 8

Ingredients:

- ✓ 1 cup rolled oats
- ✓ 1/8 teaspoon salt
- ✓ ¼ cup chocolate chips, vegan

Ingredients:

- ✓ ¼ cup maple syrup
- ✓ 1 cup peanut butter

Directions:

- ❖ Take a medium saucepan, place it over medium heat, add peanut butter, salt, and maple syrup and then whisk until combined and thickened; this will take 5 minutes.
- ❖ Remove pan from heat, place oats in a bowl, pour peanut butter mixture on it and then stir until well combined.
- ❖ Take an 8-by-6 inches baking dish, line it with a parchment sheet, spoon the oats mixture in it, and then spread evenly, pressing the mixture into the dish.

- ❖ Sprinkle the chocolate chips on top, press them into the bar mixture and then let the mixture rest in the refrigerator for 30 minutes or more until set.
- ❖ When ready to eat, cut the bar mixture into even size pieces and then serve.

170) BAKED APPLES

Preparation Time: 5 minutes   Cooking Time: 20 minutes   Servings: 4

Ingredients:

- ✓ 6 medium apples, peeled, cut into chunks
- ✓ 1 teaspoon ground cinnamon

Ingredients:

- ✓ 2 tablespoons melted coconut oil

Directions:

- ❖ Switch on the oven, then set it to 350 degrees F and let it preheat.
- ❖ Take a medium baking dish, and then spread apple pieces in it.
- ❖ Take a small bowl, place coconut oil in it, stir in cinnamon, drizzle this mixture over apples and then toss until coated.

- ❖
- ❖ Place the baking dish into the oven and then bake for 20 minutes or more until apples turn soft, stirring halfway.
- ❖ Serve straight away.

171) MIXED-FRUIT MINI PIES

Preparation Time: 15 minutes   Cooking Time: 20   minutes   Servings: 6

Ingredients:

- ✓ 1/2 cup oat flour
- ✓ 1/4 cup almond flour
- ✓ 1/2 cup chopped toasted hazelnuts
- ✓ 1/4 cup shredded coconut
- ✓ 1/3 cup coconut oil, melted
- ✓ 2tablespoons maple syrup, divided

Ingredients:

- ✓ 1/4 teaspoon salt
- ✓ 3 medium ripe peaches, peeled and chopped
- ✓ 1 cup blueberries
- ✓ 1 cup raspberries
- ✓ 1 teaspoon vanilla
- ✓ 1 tablespoon orange juice

Directions:

- ❖ Preheat oven to 400F. Grease six (1-cup) ovenproof custard cups with coconut oil and set aside.
- ❖ In a medium bowl, merge oat flour, almond flour, hazelnuts, and coconut and toss
- ❖ Add melted coconut oil, 1 tablespoon maple syrup, and salt and mix until crumbly; set aside.
- ❖ In another medium bowl, combine peaches, blueberries, and raspberries

- ❖ Sprinkle with vanilla, orange juice and remaining 1 tablespoon maple syrup and toss gently
- ❖ Divide among prepared custard cups. Top with crumble mixture.
- ❖ Set custard cups on a large rimmed baking sheet and bakes or until fruit is bubbly and tender and topping is browned.
- ❖ Serve warm or cool.

172) CRUSTLESS APPLE PIE

Preparation Time: 15 minutes   Cooking Time: 20   minutes   Servings: 8

Ingredients:

- ✓ 8 medium apples, peeled, cored, and sliced
- ✓ 3 tablespoons orange juice
- ✓ 3 tablespoons water
- ✓ 1/2 cup chopped pecans

Ingredients:

- ✓ 1/3 cup maple syrup
- ✓ 1/4 cup grass-fed butter, melted
- ✓ 1/2 teaspoon cinnamon

Directions:

- ❖ Grease a 41/2-quart slow cooker with olive oil. Arrange apple slices to cover the bottom of the slow cooker.
- ❖ In a small bowl or measuring cup, stir orange juice and water to mix. Evenly drizzle over apples.

- ❖ In another small bowl, combine pecans, maple syrup, butter, and cinnamon; mix well. Evenly crumble pecan mixture over apples.
- ❖ Seal and cook on high for 2 hours or on low for 4 hours. Serve warm or chilled.

173) APPLE DATE "CRISP"

Preparation Time: 15 minutes   Cooking Time: 4hours   Servings: 8

Ingredients:

- ✓ 6 cups cored, peeled, and thinly sliced Golden Delicious apples
- ✓ 2 teaspoons lemon juice
- ✓ 1/3 cup chopped dates
- ✓ 11/3 cups finely chopped almonds
- ✓ 1/2 cup almond flour
- ✓ 1/2 cup maple syrup

Ingredients:

- ✓ 1/2 teaspoon ground cinnamon
- ✓ 1/2 teaspoon ground ginger
- ✓ 1/8 teaspoon ground nutmeg
- ✓ 1/8 teaspoon ground cloves
- ✓ 4 tablespoons grass-fed butter

Directions:

- ❖ Combine apples, lemon juice, and dates in a large bowl, and mix well. Transfer mixture to a 41/2-quart slow cooker.
- ❖ In a separate medium bowl, combine almonds, flour, maple syrup, cinnamon, ginger, nutmeg, and cloves. Cut in grass-fed butter with two knives or a pastry blender. Sprinkle nut mixture over apples and smooth down

- ❖ Cook on low for 4 hours. Serve warm.

174) PEACH COBBLER

Preparation Time: 15 minutes   Cooking Time: 2hours   Servings: 8

Ingredients:

- ✓ 2 (16-ounce) packages frozen peaches, thawed and drained 3/4 cup maple syrup
- ✓ 2 teaspoons ground cinnamon, divided
- ✓ 1/2 teaspoon ground nutmeg

Ingredients:

- ✓ 3/4 cup almond flour
- ✓ 6 tablespoons coconut butter
- ✓ 1 fresh peach, cut into slices Sprig of mint

Directions:

- ❖ Combine peaches, 3/4 cup maple syrup, 11/2 teaspoons cinnamon, and nutmeg in a large bowl. Transfer to a 41/2-quart slow cooker.
- ❖ In a separate small bowl, combine flour with remaining 1 tablespoon maple syrup and 1/2 teaspoon cinnamon.

- ❖ Cut in coconut butter with two knives or a pastry blender and then spread mixture over peaches.
- ❖ Seal and cook on high for 2 hours. Garnish around the cobbler with fresh peaches and put a sprig of mint leaves in the center. Serve warm.

175) BLUEBERRY COCONUT CRISP

Preparation Time: 15 minutes   Cooking Time: 45 minutes   Servings: 8

Ingredients:

- ✓ 4 cups fresh blueberries
- ✓ 1/4 cup maple syrup, if needed
- ✓ 11/2 teaspoons vanilla
- ✓ 1 tablespoon lemon juice
- ✓ 1 cup chopped pecans

Ingredients:

- ✓ 1 cup unsweetened shredded coconut
- ✓ 1/3 cup coconut flour
- ✓ 3 tablespoons coconut oil
- ✓ 3 tablespoons grass-fed butter
- ✓ 1/8 teaspoon salt

Directions:

- ❖ Preheat oven to 400F. Grease an 8" square glass pan with coconut oil.
- ❖ Combine blueberries, maple syrup (if using), vanilla, and lemon juice in the pan and toss gently; set aside.

- ❖ In a medium bowl, combine pecans, coconut, and coconut flour. Add coconut oil, grass-fed butter, and salt and mix until crumbly. Sprinkle over blueberries.
- ❖ Bake for 35-40 minutes or until blueberry mixture is bubbly. Serve warm or cool.

176) PLUM BLUEBERRY COCONUT CRUMBLE

Preparation Time: 15 minutes   Cooking Time: 45 minutes   Servings: 8

Ingredients:

- ✓ 8 medium plums, stones removed, sliced
- ✓ 2 cups blueberries
- ✓ 2 tablespoons maple syrup
- ✓ 2 tablespoons lemon juice
- ✓ 1 tablespoon arrowroot powder
- ✓ 1 cup unsweetened coconut flakes

Ingredients:

- ✓ 1 cup rolled oats
- ✓ 1 cup chopped pecans
- ✓ 2/3 cup coconut flour
- ✓ 1/4 teaspoon baking soda
- ✓ 1/2 teaspoon cream of tartar
- ✓ 1/4 teaspoon salt
- ✓ 1/3 cup coconut oil, melted

Directions:

- ❖ Preheat oven to 350F. Grease a 9" square baking dish with coconut oil.
- ❖ Combine plums and blueberries in prepared dish. Drizzle with maple syrup, lemon juice, and arrowroot powder and toss to coat.
- ❖ In a medium bowl, combine coconut flakes, oats, pecans, coconut flour, baking soda, cream of tartar, and salt
- ❖ Add coconut oil and mix until crumbly. Pat mixture on top of fruit in dish.
- ❖ Bake for 40-45 minutes or until fruit is bubbly and topping is golden. Serve warm.

177) COCONUT DROPS

Preparation Time: 15 minutes   Cooking Time: 48 minutes   Servings: 8

Ingredients:

- ✓ 11/2 pounds dark chocolate, chopped

Ingredients:

- ✓ 21/2 cups unsweetened shredded coconut

Directions:

- ❖ In large heavy saucepan, melt all but 1/2 cup chocolate over low heat, stirring frequently, until melted and smooth.
- ❖ Detach pan from heat and stir in reserved chocolate. Stir constantly until mixture is smooth again.
- ❖
- ❖ Add coconut and mix well.
- ❖ Drop mounds of this mixture onto parchment paper. Let stand until set

178) BLACKBERRY COMPOTE

Preparation Time: 15 minutes   Cooking Time: 3 hours   Servings: 6

Ingredients:

- ✓ 2 cups blackberries
- ✓ 1/4 cup maple syrup

Ingredients:

- ✓ 1/4 cup water

Directions:

- ❖ Set all ingredients in a 2-quart slow cooker
- ❖ Cook on low for 3 hours, remove the lid, and cook on high for 4 hours.

179) GLUTEN-FREE FLOURLESS CHOCOLATE COOKIES

Preparation Time: 15 minutes   Cooking Time: 22 minutes   Servings: 4

Ingredients:

- ✓ 1/2 cup very dark chocolate chips 63%
- ✓ 1/2 cup chopped pecans
- ✓ 3-4 large egg whites
- ✓ 1 teaspoon vanilla extract

Ingredients:

- ✓ 1 1/2 cups Stevia
- ✓ 6 Tablespoons unsweetened cocoa powder
- ✓ 1/4 teaspoon salt

Directions:

- ❖ Heat oven to 350 degrees.
- ❖ Cover baking sheet in baking parchment and spray with cooking spray.
- ❖ In a mixing bowl, mix stevia, cocoa, salt, chocolate chips, and pecans together.
- ❖ Add vanilla with three egg whites and stir to moisten batter.
- ❖ If all the dry ingredients aren't moistened or it is too thick, add one more egg white

- ❖ (It should be very soft / sticky, but not soupy.)
- ❖ Place rounded teaspoons of dough onto cookie sheet, 2"-3" apart as cookies will spread and thin while baking.
- ❖ Bake for 11-12 minutes.
- ❖ Allow cookies to set-up on the pan for 5-8 minutes before removing to cooling rack.

180) PICO DE GALLO

Preparation Time: 15 minutes   Cooking Time: 7 minutes   Servings: 2

Ingredients:

- ✓ 1 large tomato, diced (about 11/2 cups)
- ✓ 1/2 cup chopped white onions
- ✓ 2 cloves garlic, minced
- ✓ 2 tablespoons lime juice

Ingredients:

- ✓ 2 tablespoons chopped fresh cilantro
- ✓ 1 jalapeño pepper, seeded and finely diced
- ✓ 1/2 teaspoon fine sea salt

Directions:

- ❖ Place all of the ingredients in a small bowl and stir until well combined.
- ❖ Set in an airtight container in the refrigerator for up to 5 days.

181) STUFFED DRIED FIGS

Preparation Time: 20 minutes   Cooking Time: 0 minutes   Servings: 4

Ingredients:

- • 12 dried figs
- • 2 Tbsps. thyme honey

Ingredients:

- • 2 Tbsps. sesame seeds
- • 24 walnut halves
- ❖
- ❖

Directions:

- ❖ Cut off the tough stalk ends of the figs.
- ❖ Slice open each fig.
- ❖ Stuff the fig openings with two walnut halves and close
- ❖

- ❖ Arrange the figs on a plate, drizzle with honey, and sprinkle the sesame seeds on it.
- ❖ Serve.

182) PEAR CROUSTADE

Preparation Time: 30 minutes   Cooking Time: 60 minutes   Servings: 10

Ingredients:

- 1 cup plus
- 1 tbsp. all-purpose flour, divided
- 4 ½ tbsps. sugar, divided
- 1/8 tsp salt
- 6 tbsps. unsalted butter, chilled, cut into ½ inch cubes
- 1 large-sized egg, separated

Ingredients:

- 1 1/2 tbsps. ice-cold water
- 3 firm, ripe pears (Bosc), peeled, cored, sliced into ¼ inch slices
- 1 tbsp. fresh lemon juice
- 1/3 tsp ground allspice
- 1 tsp anise seeds

Directions:

- ❖ Pour 1 cup of flour, 1 ½ Tbsps. of sugar, butter, and salt into a food processor and combine the ingredients by pulsing.
- ❖ Whisk the yolk of the egg and ice water in a separate bowl. Mix the egg mixture with the flour mixture. It will form a dough, wrap it, and set aside for an hour.
- ❖ Set the oven to 400°F.
- ❖ Mix the pear, sugar, leftover flour, allspice, anise seed, and lemon juice in a large bowl to make a filling.
- ❖ Arrange the filling on the center of the dough.
- ❖ Bake for about 40 minutes. Cool for about 15 minutes before serving.

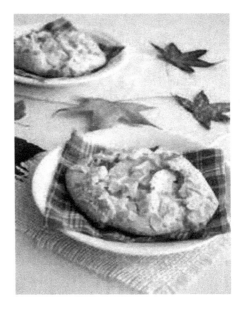

183) MELOMAKARONA

Preparation Time: 20 minutes   Cooking Time: 45 minutes   Servings: 20

Ingredients:

- 4 cups of sugar, divided
- 4 cups of water
- 1 cup plus
- 1 tbsp. honey, divided
- 1 (2-inch) strip orange peel, pith removed
- 1 cinnamon stick
- ½ cup extra-virgin olive oil
- ¼ cup unsalted butter,
- ¼ cup Metaxa brandy or any other brandy
- 1 tbsp. grated

Ingredients:

- Orange zest
- ¾ cup of orange juice
- ¼ tsp baking soda
- 3 cups pastry flour
- ¾ cup fine semolina flour
- 1 ½ tsp baking powder
- 4 tsp ground cinnamon, divided
- 1 tsp ground cloves, divided
- 1 cup finely chopped walnut
- 1/3 cup brown sugar

Directions:

- ❖ Mix 3 ½ cups of sugar, 1 cup honey, orange peel, cinnamon stick, and water in a pot and heat it for about 10 minutes.
- ❖ Mix the sugar, oil, and butter for about minutes, then add the brandy, leftover honey, and zest. Then add a mixture of baking soda and orange juice. Mix thoroughly.
- ❖ In a distinct bowl, blend the pastry flour, baking powder, semolina, 2 tsp of cinnamon, and ½ tsp. of cloves
- ❖ Add the mixture to the mixer slowly. Run the mixer until the ingredients form a dough
- ❖ Cover and set aside for 30 minutes.

- ❖ Set the oven to 350°F
- ❖ With your palms, form small oval balls from the dough. Make a total of forty balls.
- ❖ Bake the cookie balls for 30 minutes, then drop them in the prepared syrup.
- ❖ Create a mixture with the walnuts, leftover cinnamon, and cloves. Spread the mixture on the top of the baked cookies.
- ❖ Serve the cookies or store them in a closed-lid container

184) EASY BANANA DATE COOKIES

Preparation Time: 15 minutes   Cooking Time: 15 minutes   Servings: 12

Ingredients:

- 1 cup chopped pitted dates
- 1 medium banana, peeled

Ingredients:

- 1/4 teaspoon vanilla
- 13/4 cups unsweetened coconut flakes

Directions:

- ❖ Preheat oven to 375F. Cover dates in water and soak until softened. Drain.
- ❖ Process together dates, banana, and vanilla in a food processor until almost smooth. Stir in coconut flakes by hand until thick.

- ❖ Drop by generous tablespoonful's onto a cookie sheet. Bake until golden brown. Cookies will be soft and chewy.

185)CRANBERRY APPLE COMPOTE

Preparation Time: 15 minutes   Cooking Time: 15 minutes   Servings: 6

Ingredients:

- 4 cups peeled, cored, sliced apples
- 1/2 cup sliced cranberries
- 1/3 cup maple syrup
- 2 tablespoons coconut oil

Ingredients:

- 1 teaspoon ground cinnamon
- 1/4 teaspoon ground nutmeg
- 3/4 cup combined chopped walnuts and almonds

Directions:

- ❖ Combine all ingredients except nuts in a 3-4-quart slow cooker.
- ❖ Cover and cook on high for 11/2-2 hours or until apples are tender.

- ❖ Sprinkle each serving with nuts

186)CHOCOLATE "GRAHAM" CRACKER BARS

Preparation Time: 15 minutes   Cooking Time: 15 minutes   Servings: 16

Ingredients:

- 1 cup finely chopped walnuts
- 1cup unsweetened grated coconut
- 3 cups crushed "Graham" Crackers

Ingredients:

- 2/3 cup canned full-fat coconut milk
- 14 ounces chopped dark chocolate
- 2 teaspoons vanilla

Directions:

- ❖ Set a 9" square pan with coconut oil and set aside. In a large bowl, combine walnuts, coconut, and cracker crumbs; set aside.
- ❖ In medium saucepan, combine coconut milk and chocolate. Melt over low heat, stirring frequently, until smooth. Stir in vanilla. Reserve 1/3 cup of this mixture.

- ❖
- ❖ Set remaining chocolate mixture over crumb mixture and stir to coat.
- ❖ Press crumb mixture into prepared pan and spread reserved chocolate over top. Place in refrigerator until set; cut into eight squares to serve.

187)HEAVENLY COOKIE BARS

Preparation Time: 15 minutes   Cooking Time: 15 minutes   Servings: 48

Ingredients:

- 2 cups maple syrup
- 4 cups almond flour
- 1/2 teaspoon nutmeg

Ingredients:

- 1/2 teaspoon ginger
- 1/2 cup dates, chopped 2 cups ground walnuts
- 1/2 cup raisins

Directions:

- ❖ Preheat oven to 350F. Set two large baking sheets with parchment paper.
- ❖ Warm maple syrup in a medium saucepan over low heat for 5 minutes and let cool slightly.

- ❖ In a bowl, sift together flour, nutmeg, and ginger. Add maple syrup and stir until well blended. Stir in dates, walnuts, and raisins.
- ❖ Roll dough to 1/4" thick and cut into forty-eight squares. Place squares on prepared baking sheets and bake for 10 minutes. Remove to rack to cool.

188) WALNUT-STUFFED SLOW-COOKED APPLES

Preparation Time: 15 minutes   Cooking Time: 4 hours   Servings: 4

Ingredients:

- 1/4 cup coarsely chopped walnuts
- 3 tablespoons dried currants
- 3/4 teaspoon ground cinnamon, divided

Ingredients:

- 4 medium Granny Smith apples, cored
- 1 cup maple syrup
- 3/4 cup apple cider

Directions:

- ❖ In a small bowl, combine walnuts and currants. Add 1/4 teaspoon cinnamon, stirring to combine.
- ❖ Place apples in a 2-quart or smaller slow cooker. Spoon walnut mixture into the cavity of each apple.
- ❖ In a medium mixing bowl, combine remaining 1/2 teaspoon cinnamon, maple syrup, and apple cider, stirring to combine. Pour over apples in the slow cooker.

- ❖ Cover and cook on low for 23/4 hours. Remove apples with a slotted spoon.
- ❖ Spoon 1/4 cup cooking liquid over each serving.

189) HEAVENLY COOKIE BARS

Preparation Time: 15 minutes   Cooking Time: 15   minutes   Servings: 48

Ingredients:

- 2 cups maple syrup
- 4 cups almond flour
- 1/2 teaspoon nutmeg

Ingredients:

- 1/2 teaspoon ginger
- 1/2 cup dates, chopped 2 cups ground walnuts

1/2 cup raisins

Directions:

- ❖ Preheat oven to 350F. Set two large baking sheets with parchment paper.
- ❖ Warm maple syrup in a medium saucepan over low heat for 5 minutes and let cool slightly.

- ❖ In a bowl, sift together flour, nutmeg, and ginger. Add maple syrup and stir until well blended. Stir in dates, walnuts, and raisins.
- ❖ Roll dough to 1/4" thick and cut into forty-eight squares. Place squares on prepared baking sheets and bake for 10 minutes. Remove to rack to cool.

190) WALNUT-STUFFED SLOW-COOKED APPLES

Preparation Time: 15 minutes   Cooking Time: 4 hours   Servings: 4

Ingredients:

- 1/4 cup coarsely chopped walnuts
- 3 tablespoons dried currants
- 3/4 teaspoon ground cinnamon, divided

Ingredients:

- 4 medium Granny Smith apples, cored
- 1 cup maple syrup
- 3/4 cup apple cider

Directions:

- ❖ In a small bowl, combine walnuts and currants. Add 1/4 teaspoon cinnamon, stirring to combine.
- ❖ Place apples in a 2-quart or smaller slow cooker. Spoon walnut mixture into the cavity of each apple.
- ❖ In a medium mixing bowl, combine remaining 1/2 teaspoon cinnamon, maple syrup, and apple cider, stirring to combine. Pour

- ❖ Cover and cook on low for 23/4 hours. Remove apples with a slotted spoon.
- ❖ Spoon 1/4 cup cooking liquid over each serving.

over apples in the slow cooker.

191) CARROT ENERGY BALLS WITH COCONUT

Preparation Time: 10 minutes   Cooking Time: 0 minutes   Servings: 4

Ingredients:

- 2 carrots, peeled, grated
- 4 teaspoons coconut shred
- 4 pecans, chopped

Ingredients:

- 4 tablespoons coconut flour
- 4 teaspoons honey
- 1 tablespoon almond flour

Directions:

- ❖ Put the grated carrot in the bowl.
- ❖ Add chopped pecans, coconut flour, almond flour, and honey.
- ❖ Stir the mixture until smooth with the help of the fork.
- ❖ Then make the small balls from the mixture and coat them in the coconut shred.

192) STRAWBERRY ICE CREAM

Preparation Time: 1 hour   Cooking Time: 10 minutes   Servings: 2

Ingredients:

- 1 cup strawberries
- 1 avocado, peeled, pitted

Ingredients:

- 1 tablespoon raw honey

Directions:

- ❖ Chop the avocado and blend it until smooth.
- ❖ Then add strawberries and blend the mixture for 2 minutes.
- ❖ After this, add raw honey and pulse it for 30 seconds.
- ❖ Put the mixture in the plastic vessel and freeze it for 1 hour. Stir it every 10 minutes.

193) PUMPKIN PIE CHIA PUDDING JARS

Preparation Time: 10 minutes   Cooking Time: 8 minutes   Servings: 4

Ingredients:

- 1 teaspoon pumpkin pie spices
- 4 tablespoons chia seeds
- 1 cup coconut cream

Ingredients:

- ¼ cup of water
- 4 teaspoons raw honey

Directions:

- ❖ In the mixing bowl mix up pumpkin pie spices, chia seeds, coconut cream, and water.
- ❖ Then transfer the mixture in the saucepan and bring it to boil.
- ❖ Remove the mixture from the heat and transfer in the serving glasses.
- ❖ Cool the pudding to the room temperature and top with raw honey.

194)CINNAMON COFFEE CAKE

Preparation Time: 15 minutes   Cooking Time: 30 minutes   Servings: 6

Ingredients:

- 1 egg, beaten
- 1 tablespoon organic almond milk
- ½ teaspoon lime juice
- 1 teaspoon coconut oil
- 2 tablespoons coconut sugar
- 1 cup almonds, blanched

Ingredients:

- 1 cup almond flour
- 1 teaspoon vanilla extract
- 1 teaspoon ground cinnamon
- 1 teaspoon flax meal
- ½ cup coconut cream

Directions:

- ❖ In the mixing bowl mix up egg, almond milk, lime juice, coconut oil, coconut sugar, almonds, almond flour, vanilla extract, ground cinnamon, and flax meal.
- ❖ Stir the mixture until it is smooth.
- ❖ After this, line the round baking pan with cinnamon mixture and flatten it if needed.

- ❖ Bake the cake for 30 minutes at 350F.
- ❖ Then cool the cake well and cut into 2 parts.
- ❖ Spread every cake part with coconut cream and sandwich them.

195)GINGERBREAD BARS

Preparation Time: 15 minutes   Cooking Time: 20 minutes   Servings: 6

Ingredients:

- 1 cup coconut flour
- 1 teaspoon ground ginger
- 1 teaspoon ground cinnamon
- ¼ teaspoon ground cardamom
- ½ teaspoon ground clove
- ¼ teaspoon salt

Ingredients:

- 2 eggs, beaten
- 2 tablespoons coconut oil, softened
- 1 teaspoon baking powder
- 2 tablespoons flax meal
- ½ cup almond flour
- 3 tablespoons raw honey

Directions:

- ❖ In the mixing bowl mix up coconut flour, ground ginger, cinnamon, cardamom, ground clove, salt, eggs, softened coconut oil, baking powder, flax meal, almond flour, and raw honey.
- ❖ Knead the smooth dough.
- ❖ After this, place it in the baking paper and flatten with the help of the rolling pin or fingertips.
- ❖ Cut the dough into the bars.

- ❖ Preheat the oven to 350F.
- ❖ Place the gingerbread bars in the oven and cook them for 20 minutes.
- ❖ Then cool the cooked dessert to the room temperature.

196)PEAR BUTTER

Preparation Time: 10 minutes   Cooking Time: 10 minutes   Servings: 2

Ingredients:

- 1 pear, peeled, chopped
- 2 tablespoons raw honey

Ingredients:

- 1 tablespoon almond butter
- 1 teaspoon ground nutmeg

Directions:

- ❖ Put the pear in the saucepan and add almond butter.
- ❖ Add ground nutmeg and bring the mixture to boil.
- ❖ After this, use the immersion blender to blend the pear mixture.

- ❖ Remove it from the heat and add honey.
- ❖ Stir it well and transfer in the glass jar.

197) GRAHAM CRACKERS

Preparation Time: 15 minutes   Cooking Time: 16 minutes   Servings: 6

Ingredients:

- 1 cup almond meal
- ½ teaspoon baking powder
- 1 tablespoon raw honey
- 1 tablespoon coconut oil, melted

Ingredients:

- ½ teaspoon vanilla extract
- ½ teaspoon ground cinnamon
- 1 oz egg, beaten

Directions:

- ❖ In the mixing bowl mix up an almond meal, baking powder, honey, coconut oil, vanilla extract, ground cinnamon, and egg.
- ❖ Knead the dough.
- ❖ Line the baking tray with baking paper.
- ❖ After this, put the cracker dough in the baking tray and flatten it with the help of the rolling pin.
- ❖ Cut the dough on the crackers and bake at 355F for 16 minutes or until the crackers get light brown edges.

198) SWEET WALNUT CLUSTERS

Preparation Time: 20 minutes   Cooking Time: 5 minutes   Servings: 4

Ingredients:

- ½ cup walnuts
- 2 teaspoons cocoa powder
- 1 tablespoon almond butter

Ingredients:

- 1 tablespoon coconut oil, melted
- 1 teaspoon vanilla extract
- 1 tablespoon raw honey

Directions:

- ❖ In the saucepan mix up cocoa powder, almond butter, coconut oil, vanilla extract, and raw honey.
- ❖ Melt the mixture but don't boil it.
- ❖ Then line the baking tray with baking paper.
- ❖ Add the walnuts in the melted cocoa mixture.
- ❖ After this, make the walnut clusters with the help of the spoon and place them in the baking tray.
- ❖ Cool the clusters well.

199) ESPRESSO BROWNIE

Preparation Time: 10 minutes   Cooking Time: 25 minutes   Servings: 4

Ingredients:

- ¼ cup brewed coffee
- 1 tablespoon cocoa powder
- ½ cup almond flour

Ingredients:

- 3 eggs, beaten
- 1 tablespoon raw honey
- 1 teaspoon coconut oil, melted

Directions:

- ❖ In the mixing bowl whisk together brewed coffee and cocoa powder.
- ❖ Then add almond flour, eggs, honey, and coconut oil.
- ❖ Stir the mixture until you get the smooth batter.
- ❖ Then line the baking tray with the baking paper.
- ❖ Pour the brownie batter in the tray and flatten it.
- ❖ Bake the brownie for 25 minutes at 350F.
- ❖ Then cool it well and cut into bars.

200)PUMPKIN SEEDS BARS

Preparation Time: 15 minutes   Cooking Time: 0 minutes   Servings: 6

Ingredients:

- ½ cup pumpkin seeds, chopped
- ¼ cup dates, chopped
- 1 tablespoon coconut oil, melted

Ingredients:

- 1 tablespoon poppy seeds
- 1 teaspoon raw honey

Directions:

- ❖ Blend the dates until smooth and put them in the mixing bowl.
- ❖ Add chopped pumpkin seeds, coconut oil, poppy seeds, and honey.
- ❖ Stir the mixture until homogenous.
- ❖ After this, put the date mixture in the baking paper and flatten it.
- ❖ Cut the mixture into the bars.

Thanks for reading this book

CPSIA information can be obtained
at www.ICGtesting.com
Printed in the USA
LVHW061754200621
690717LV00008B/367